STUDENT WORKBOOK FOR

ILLUSTRATED

Dental Embryology, Histology, AND Anatomy

T0294744

STUDENT WORKBOOK FOR

ILLUSTRATED

Dental Embryology, Histology, AND Anatomy

FIFTH EDITION

MARGARET J. FEHRENBACH, RDH, MS

Oral Biologist and Dental Hygienist,
Adjunct Instructor, Bachelor of Applied Science Degree Dental Hygiene Program,
Seattle Central College, Seattle, Washington
Educational Consultant and Dental Science Technical Writer,
Seattle, Washington

ELSEVIER

Elsevier
3251 Riverport Lane
St. Louis, Missouri 63043

STUDENT WORKBOOK FOR ILLUSTRATED DENTAL EMBRYOLOGY,   ISBN: 978-0-323-63990-3
HISTOLOGY, AND ANATOMY, FIFTH EDITION

Notice

Practitioners and researchers must always rely on their own experience and knowledge in evaluating and
using any information, methods, compounds or experiments described herein. Because of rapid advances
in the medical sciences, in particular, independent verification of diagnoses and drug dosages should
be made. To the fullest extent of the law, no responsibility is assumed by Elsevier, authors, editors or
contributors for any injury and/or damage to persons or property as a matter of products liability,
negligence or otherwise, or from any use or operation of any methods, products, instructions, or ideas
contained in the material herein.

Content Strategist: Joslyn Dumas
Senior Content Development Manager: Luke Held
Senior Content Development Specialist: Kelly Skelton
Publishing Services Manager: Shereen Jameel
Senior Project Manager: Kamatchi Madhavan
Cover Designer: Gopalakrishnan Venkatraman

Printed in the United States of America

Last digit is the print number: 9 8 7 6 5 4

Working together
to grow libraries in
developing countries

www.elsevier.com • www.bookaid.org

PREFACE

This companion to *Illustrated Dental Embryology, Histology, and Anatomy* provides a wide range of activities and skill-building exercises to strengthen the student dental professional's understanding of the principles discussed in the main textbook. This workbook features activities such as structure identification exercises, glossary exercises, tooth-drawing exercises, infection control guidelines for extracted teeth, and review questions. Also included are patient examination procedures for extraoral and intraoral structures, the dentition, and occlusal evaluation in order to integrate the clinical information with the basic science information within these included clinical exercises. Case studies are also included as well as removable flashcards using the original illustrations of the permanent dentition from the textbook.

Additional material for students can be found online on the associated Evolve website. We hope that this material will help students integrate their knowledge more easily into clinical dental coursework.

Margaret J. Fehrenbach, RDH, MS, Editor

CONTENTS

STUDENT WORKBOOK FOR

ILLUSTRATED

Dental Embryology, Histology, AND Anatomy

Note: Answers can be obtained from comparing your fill-ins to the labels on numbered figures from the textbook. Feel free to add additional labeling as needed and other notations.

UNIT I: OROFACIAL STRUCTURE

Chapter 1: Face and Neck Regions

1. Figure 1.1

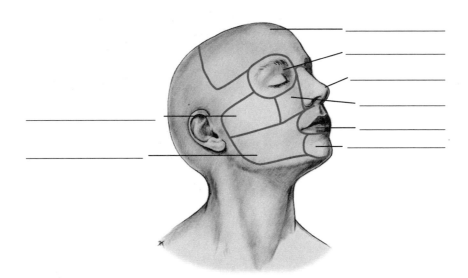

2. Figure 1.11

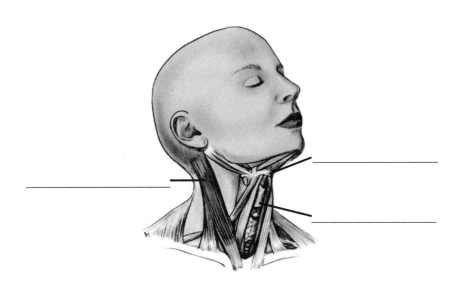

3. Figure 1.2, *A, B*

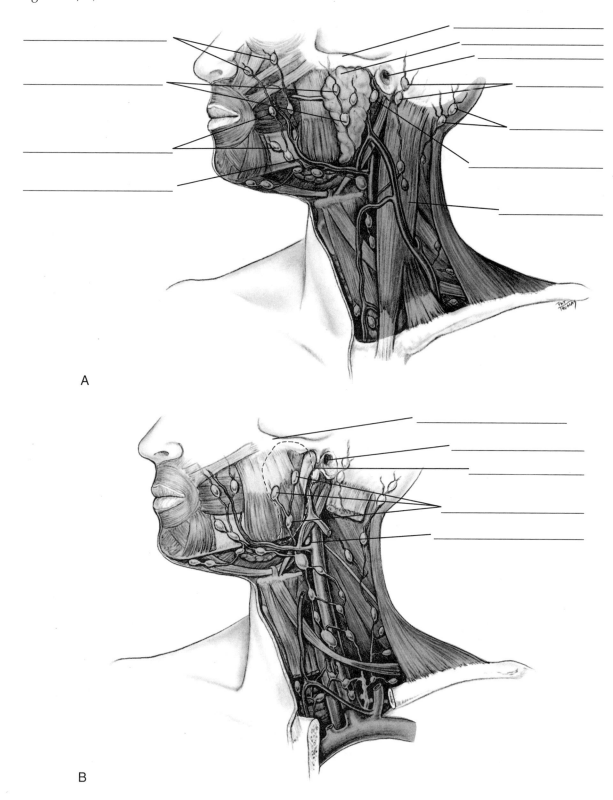

A

B

4. Figure 1.5

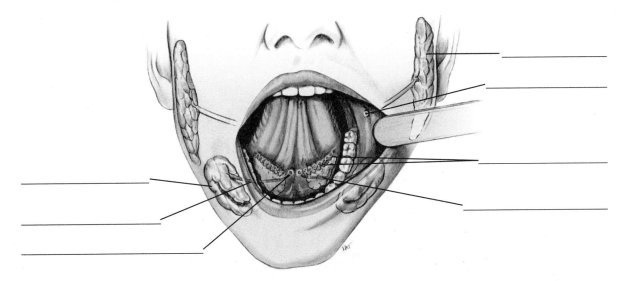

5. Figure 1.13

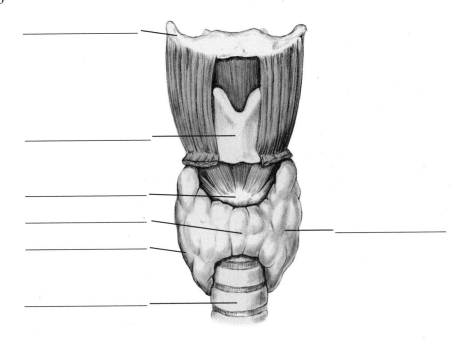

6. Figure 1.12, *A, B*

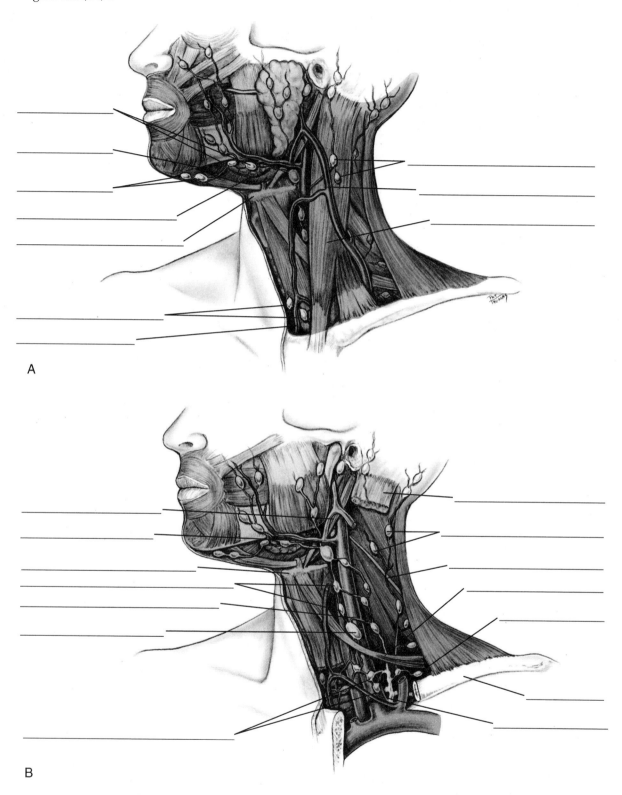

A

B

Chapter 2: Oral Cavity and Pharynx

7. Figure 2.1

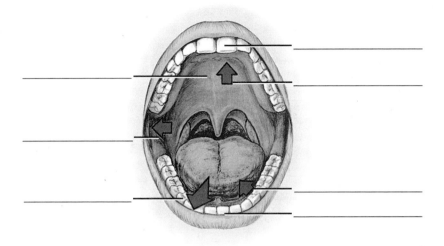

8. Figure 2.4

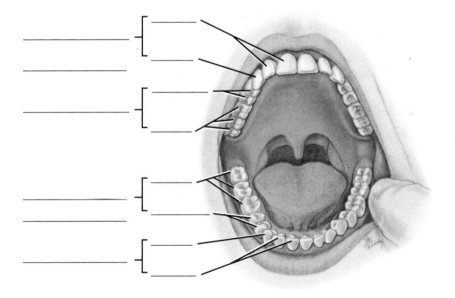

9. Figure 2.6

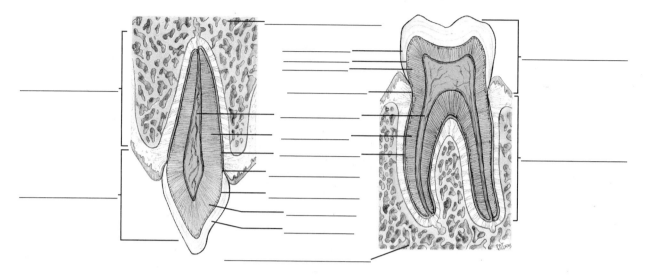

10. Figure 2.11

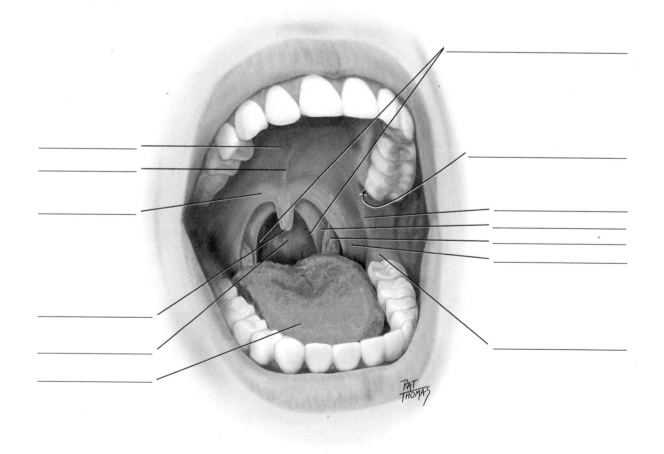

11. Figure 2.14, *A*

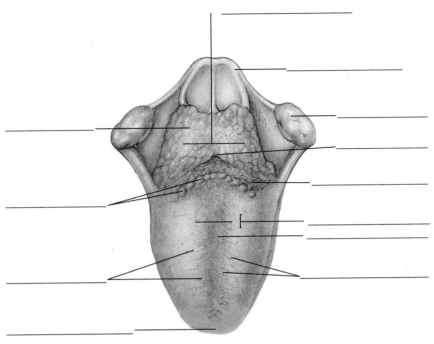

12. Figure 2.18

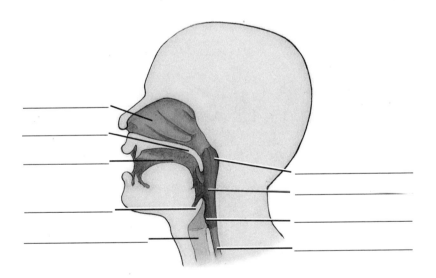

UNIT II: DENTAL EMBRYOLOGY

Chapter 3: Prenatal Development

1. Figure 3.4, *B*

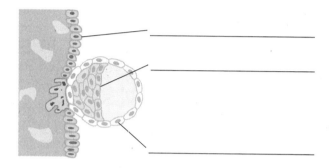

2. Figure 3.6, *A*

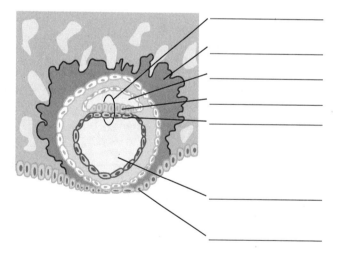

3. Figure 3.7

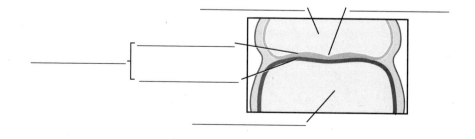

4. Figure 3.8

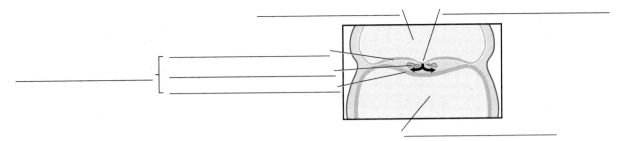

5. Figure 3.9

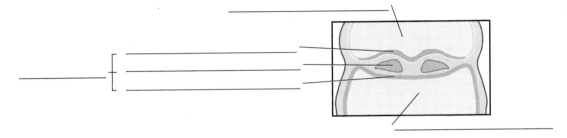

6. Figure 3.10, *A, B, C*

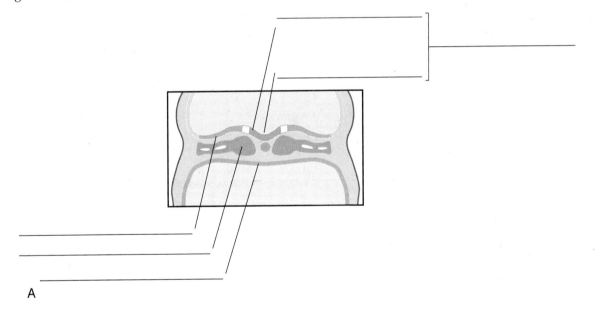

A

6. Figure 3.10, *A, B, C* (continued)

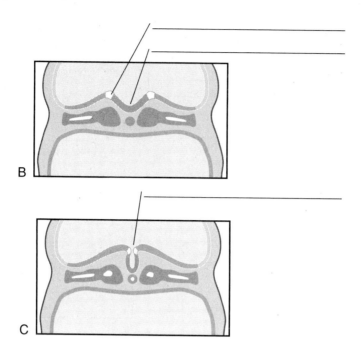

7. Figure 3.12, *A, B*

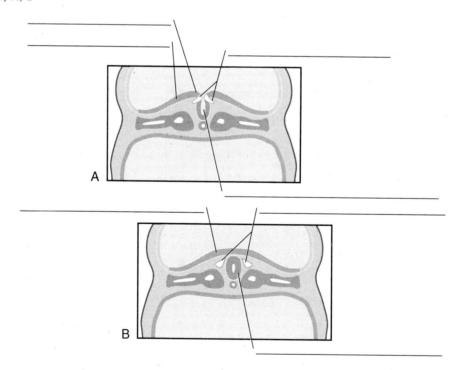

8. Figure 3.14, *B, C*

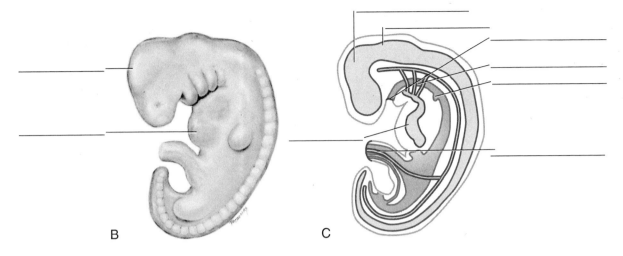

B   C

Chapter 4: Face and Neck Development

9. Figure 4.2

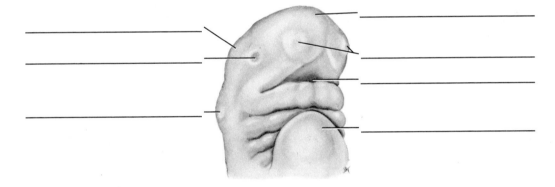

10. Figure 4.3

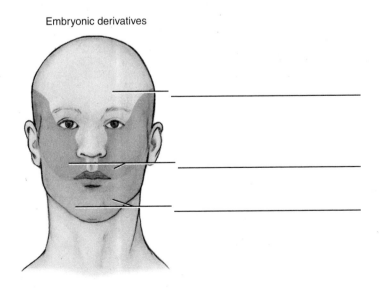

Embryonic derivatives

11. Figure 4.5

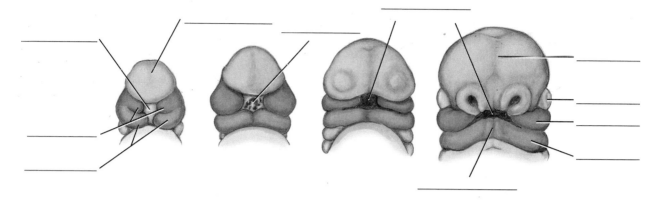

12. Figure 4.6

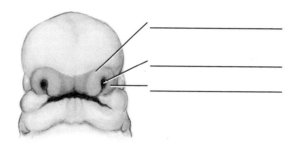

13. Figure 4.7, *B, C*

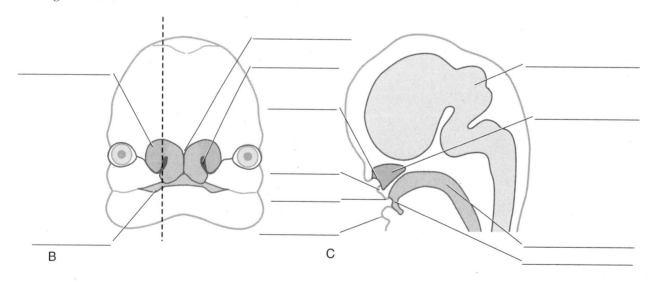

B   C

14. Figure 4.11, *B, C*

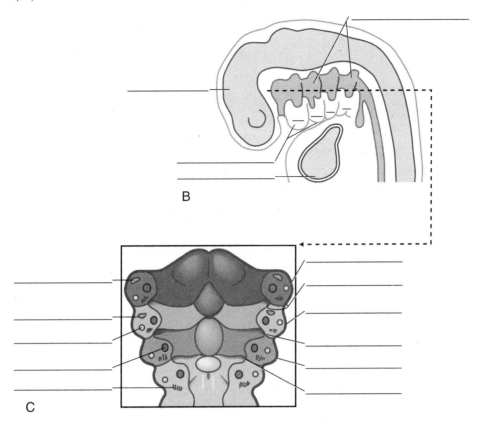

B

C

Chapter 5: Orofacial Development

15. Figure 5.1, *A, B*

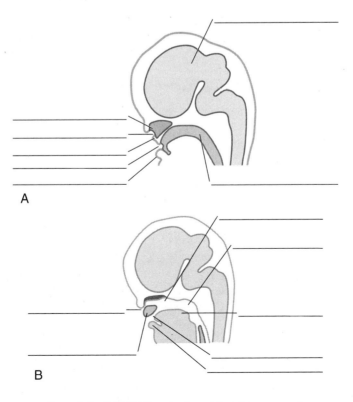

A

B

16. Figure 5.2, *A, C*

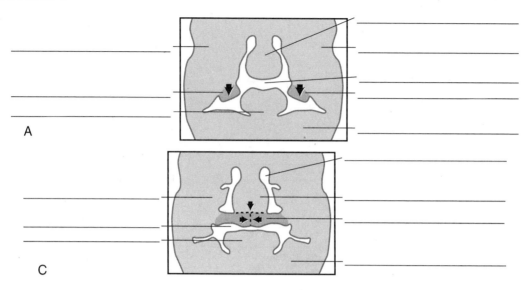

17. Figure 5.4, *B, C, D*

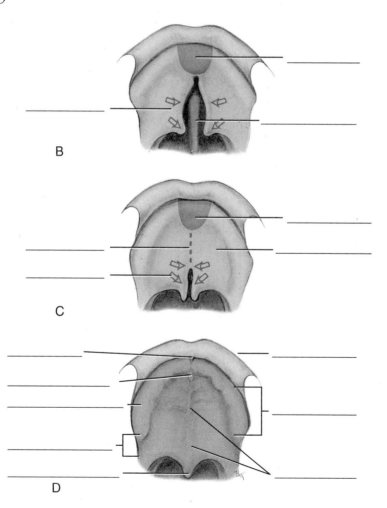

18. Figure 5.9, *A, B, C*

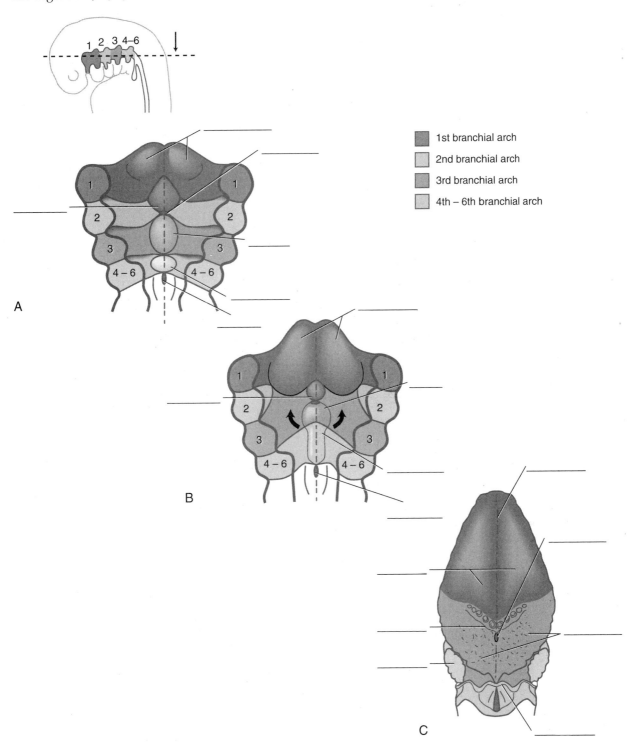

1st branchial arch

2nd branchial arch

3rd branchial arch

4th – 6th branchial arch

Chapter 6: Tooth Development and Eruption

19. Figure 6.2

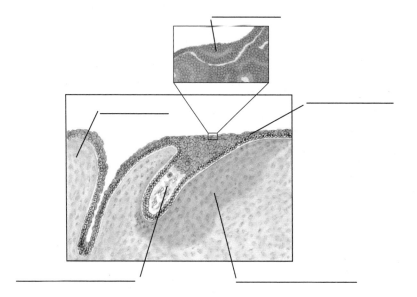

20. Figure 6.3

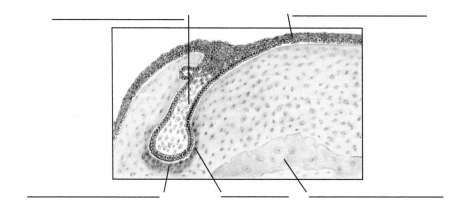

21. Figure 6.5

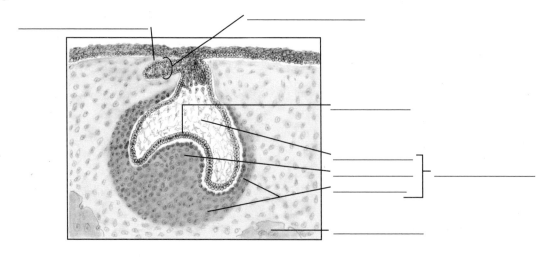

22. Figure 6.7

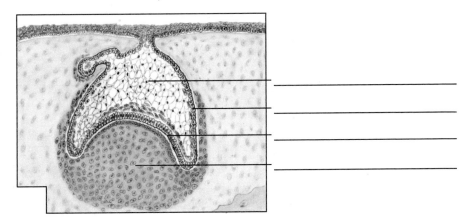

23. Figure 6.7

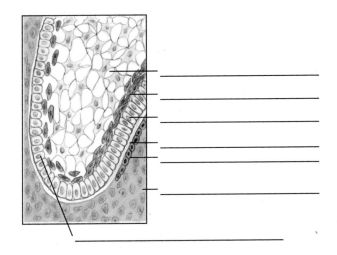

24. Figure 6.12

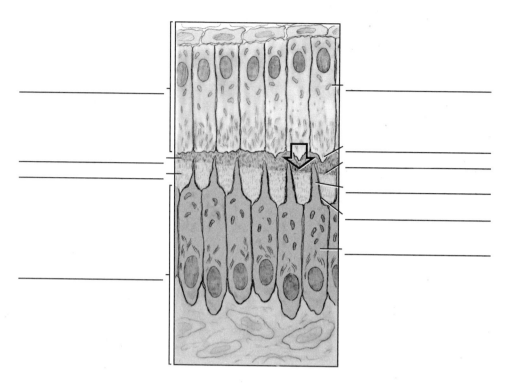

25. Figure 6.13

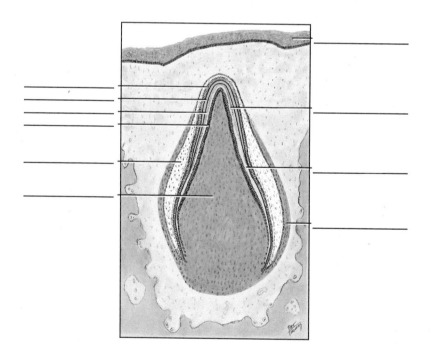

26. Figure 6.18, *A, B*

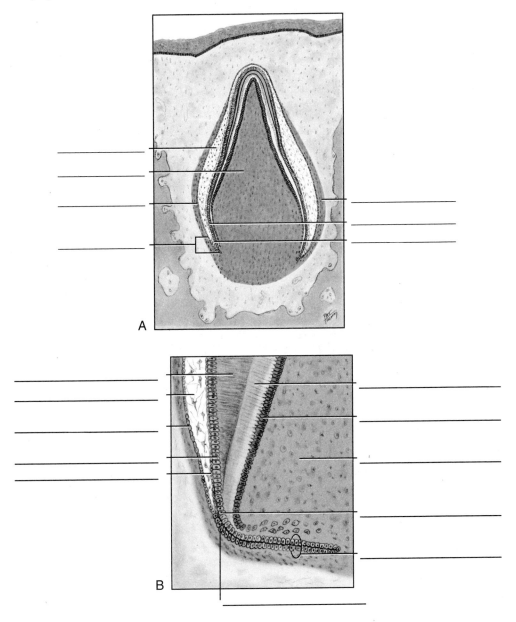

A

B

27. Figure 6.19

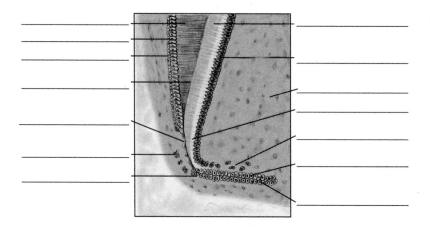

28. Figure 6.20

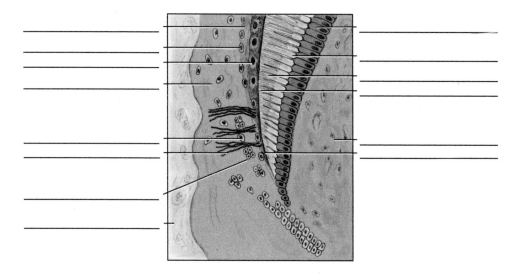

29. Figure 6.23

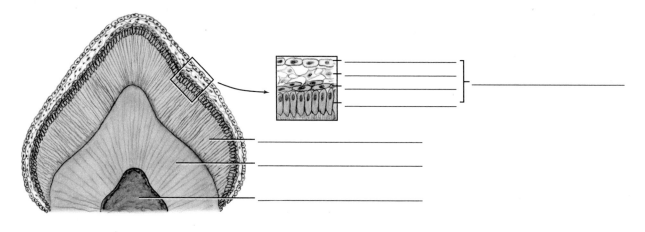

30. Figure 6.26

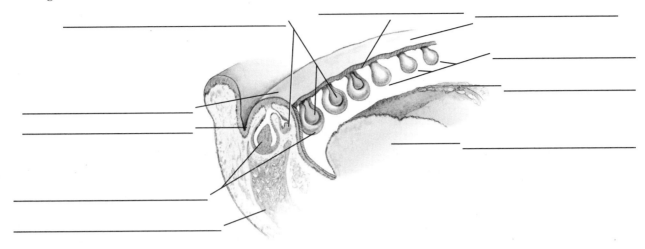

31. Figure 6.27, *B*, *C* (Courtesy Margaret J. Fehrenbach, RDH, MS.)

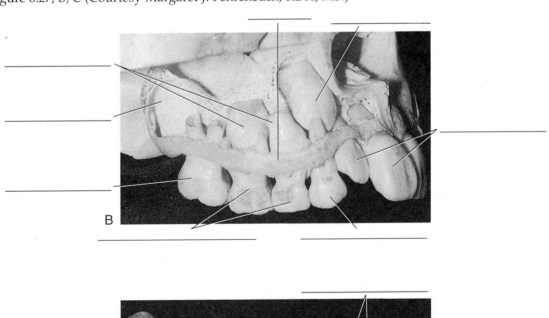

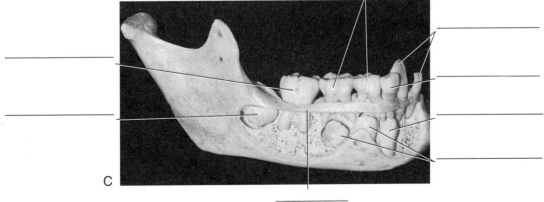

UNIT III: DENTAL HISTOLOGY

Chapter 7: Cells

1. Figure 7.2

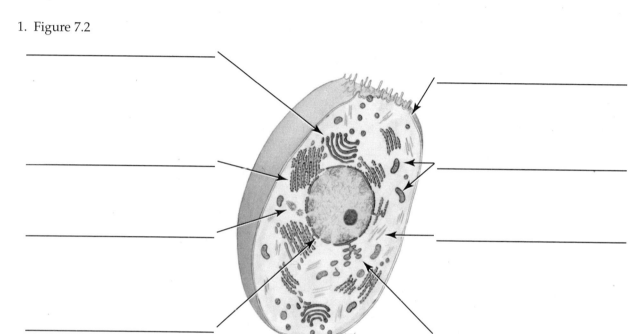

2. Figure 7.3

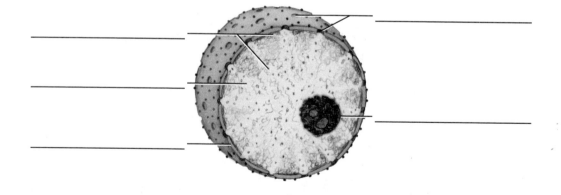

Chapter 8: Basic Tissue

3. Figure 8.4

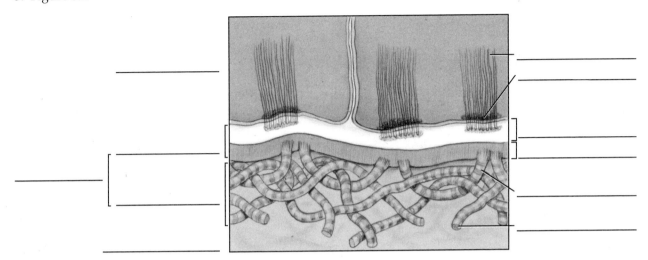

4. Figure 8.5, *A*

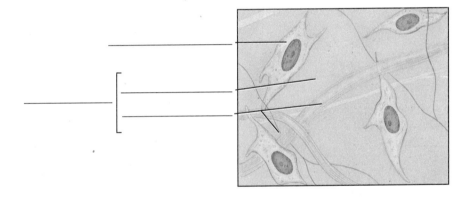

5. Figure 8.6

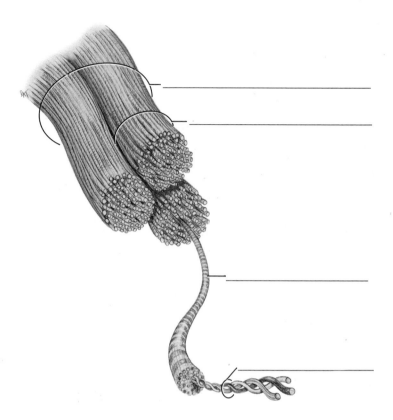

6. Figure 8.7

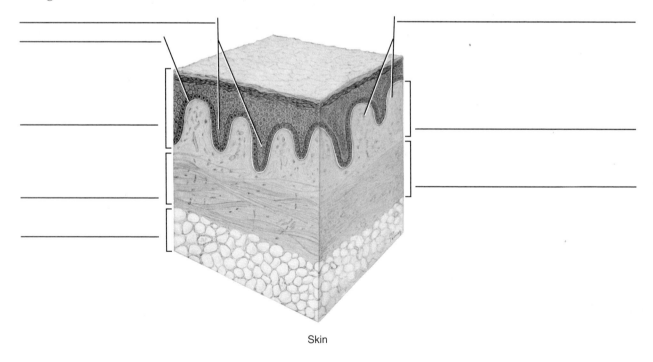

Skin

7. Figure 8.8

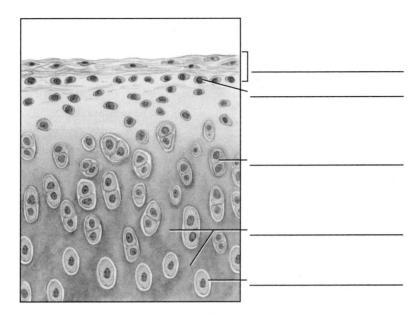

8. Figure 8.9

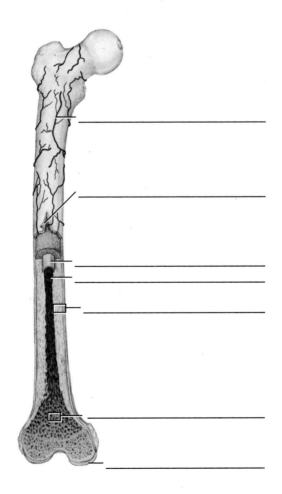

9. Figure 8.10

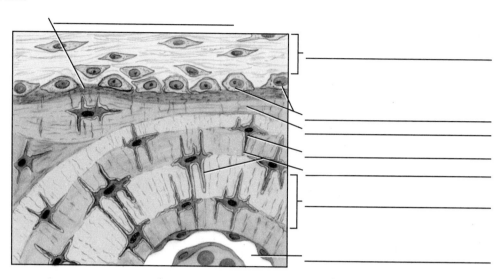

10. Figure 8.11, *A* (From Applegate EJ. *The Anatomy and Physiology Learning System.* 4th ed. St. Louis: Elsevier; 2011.)

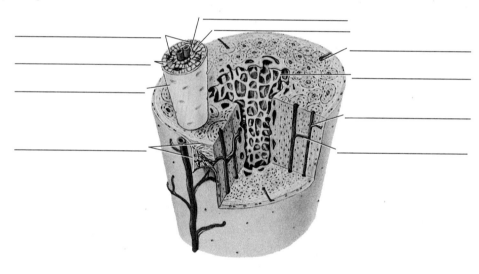

11. Figure 8.15

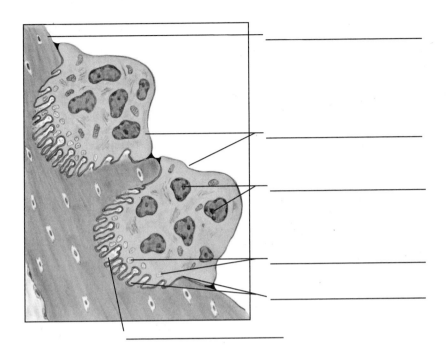

_____

_____

_____

_____

_____

_____

12. Figure 8.18

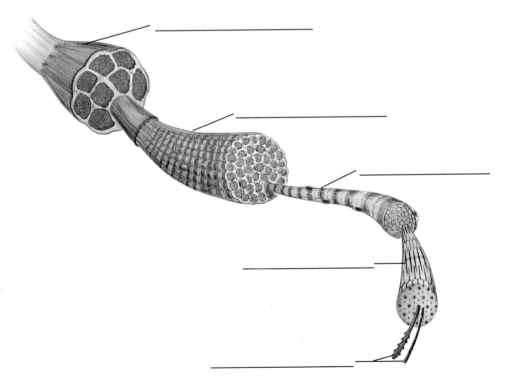

_____

_____

_____

_____

_____

13. Figure 8.19

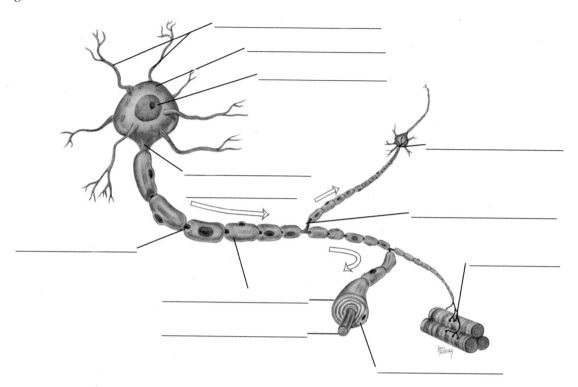

Chapter 9: Oral Mucosa

14. Figure 9.1

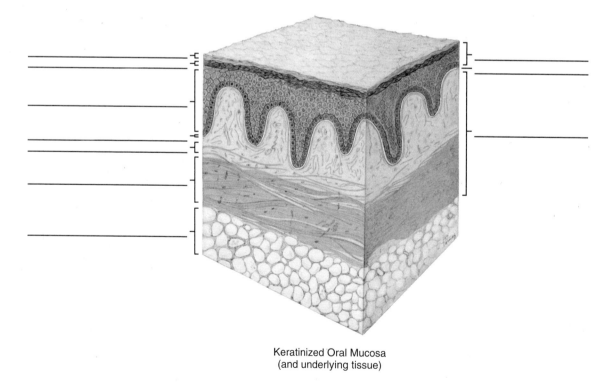

Keratinized Oral Mucosa
(and underlying tissue)

15. Figure 9.2

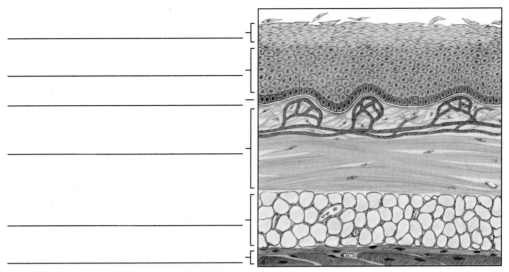

Nonkeratinized Stratified Squamous Epithelium
(and deeper tissue)

16. Figure 9.3

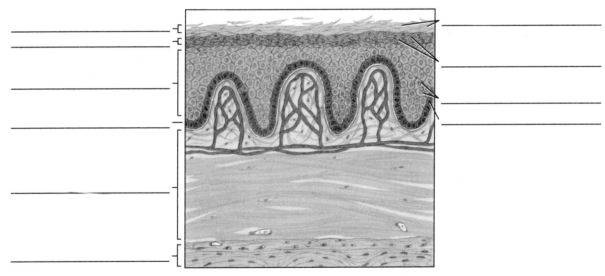

Orthokeratinized Stratified Squamous Epithelium
(and deeper tissue)

17. Figure 9.5

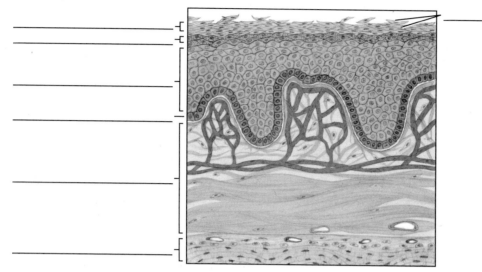

Parakeratinized Stratified Squamous Epithelium
(and deeper tissue)

18. Figure 9.6

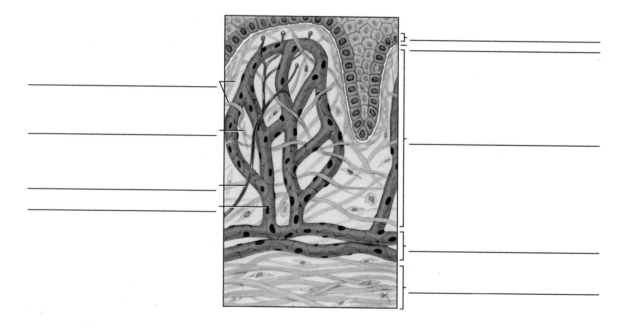

19. Figure 9.13

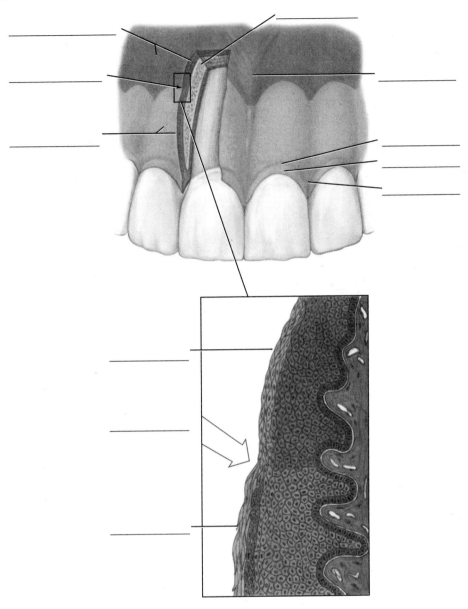

20. Figure 9.17

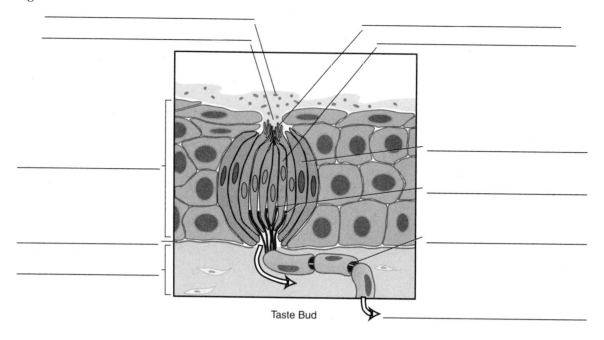

Taste Bud

Chapter 10: Gingival and Dentogingival Junctional Tissue

21. Figure 10.1

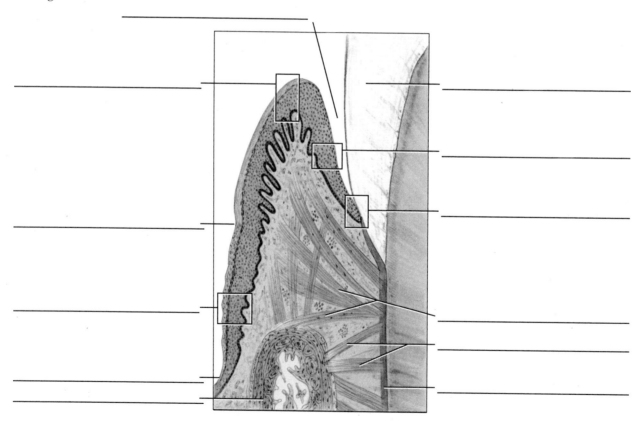

22. Figure 10.6

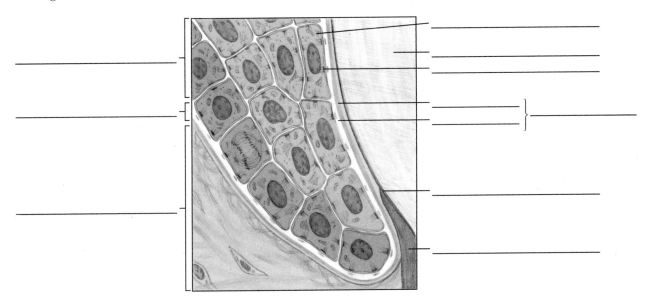

Chapter 11: Head and Neck Structures

23. Figure 11.1, *B*

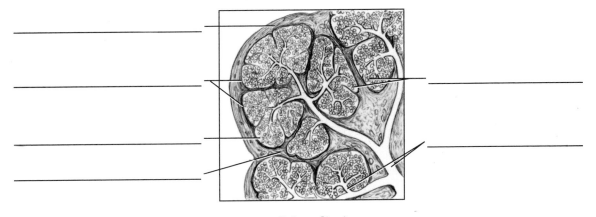

Salivary Gland

24. Figure 11.6

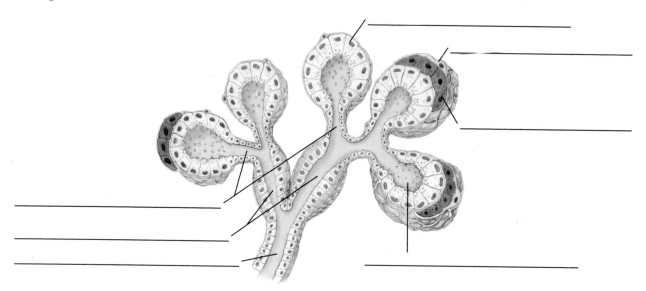

25. Figure 11.7, *A, B, C*

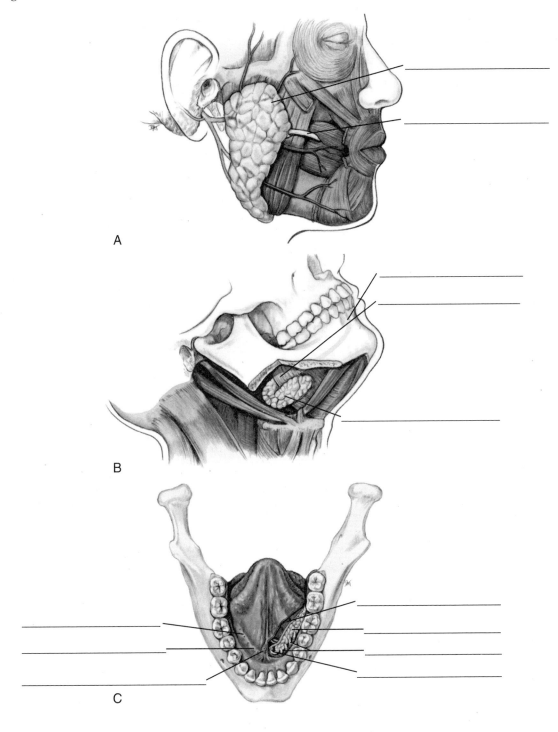

A

B

C

26. Figure 11.13, *B*

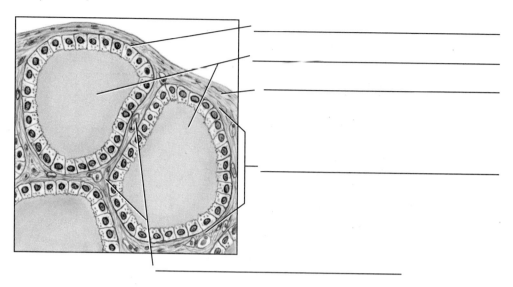

27. Figure 11.16, *A*

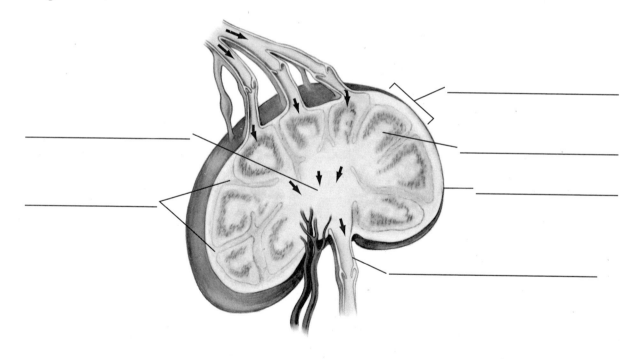

28. Figure 11.17, *A*

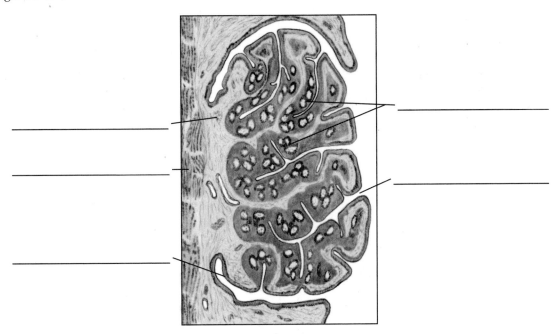

29. Figure 11.19

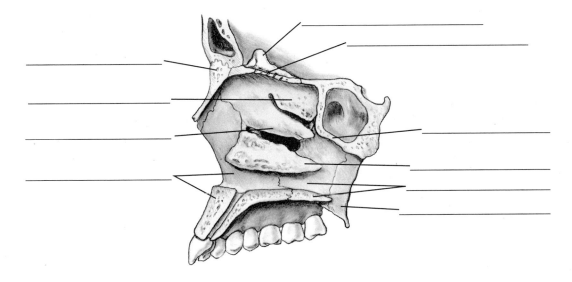

30. Figure 11.20

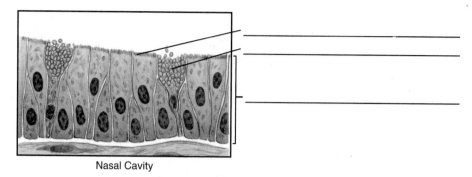

Nasal Cavity

31. Figure 11.21

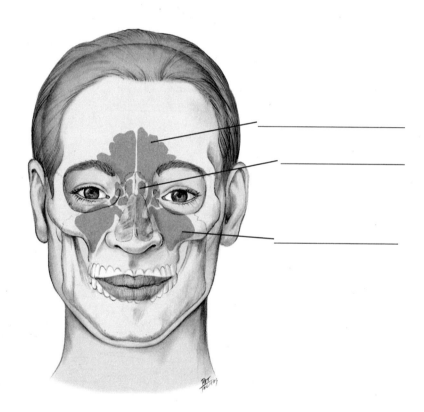

Chapter 12: Enamel

32. Figure 12.4, *A*, *B*, Figure 12.6, *A*

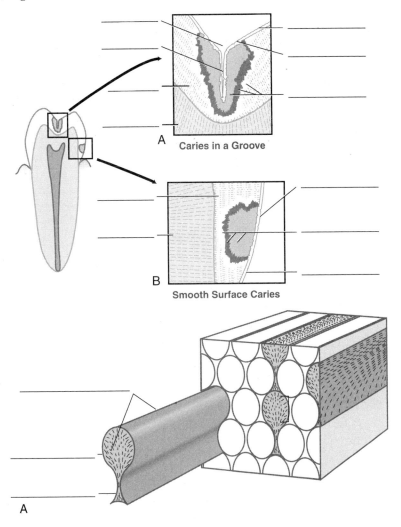

Chapter 13: Dentin and Pulp

33. Figure 13.9, Figure 13.16, *B*

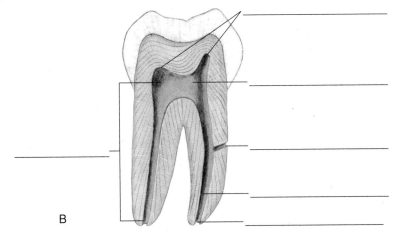

Chapter 14: Periodontium: Cementum, Alveolar Process, and Periodontal Ligament

34. Figure 14.1

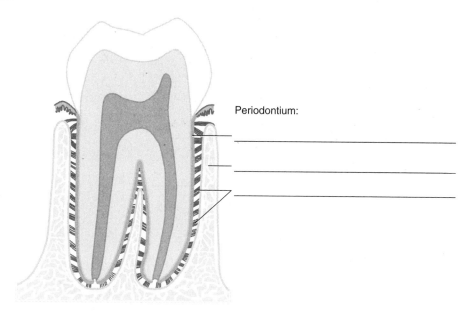

Periodontium:

35. Figure 14.2

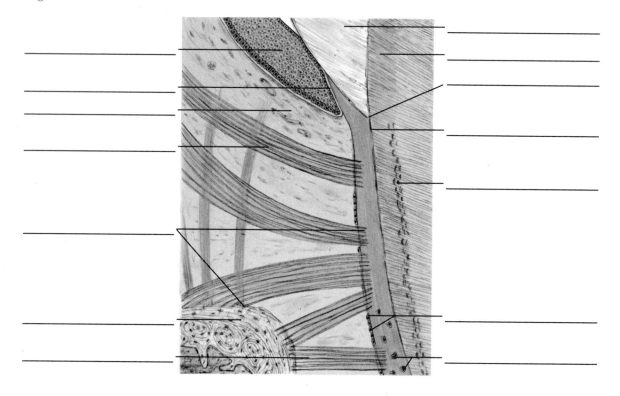

36. Figure 14.14, *A, B, C* (Courtesy Margaret J. Fehrenbach, RDH, MS.)

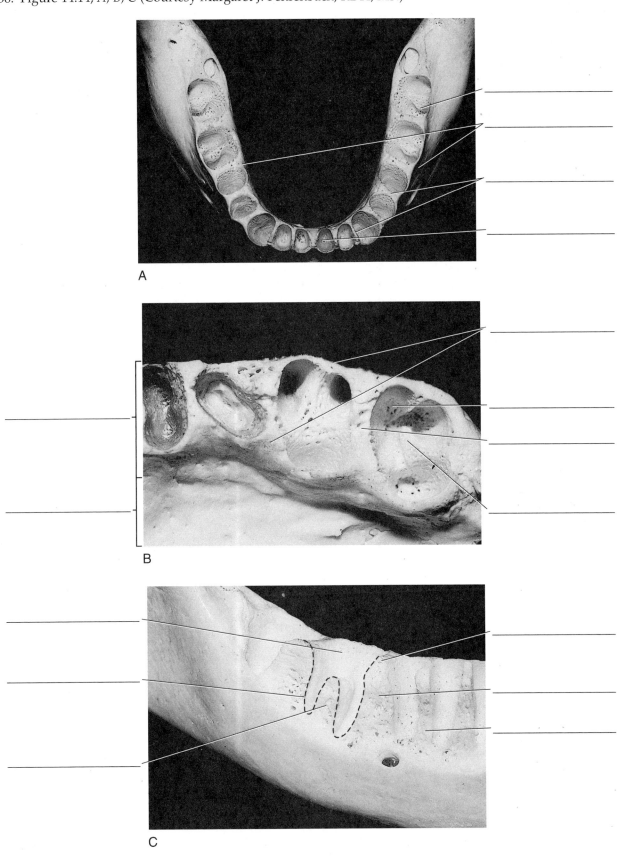

37. Figure 14.20

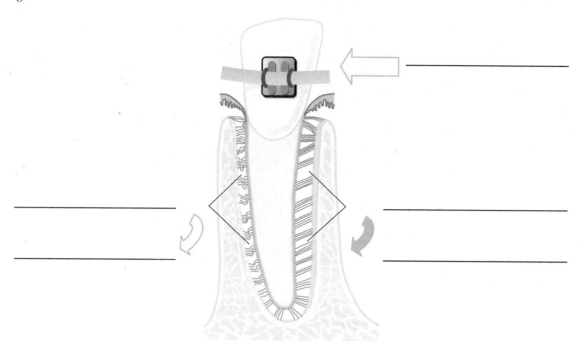

Orthodontic Tooth Movement

38. Figure 14.27

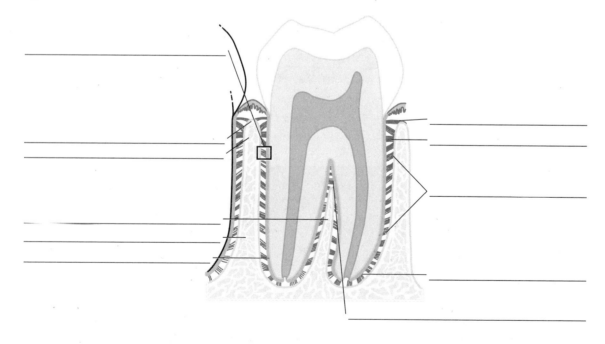

39. Figure 14.31

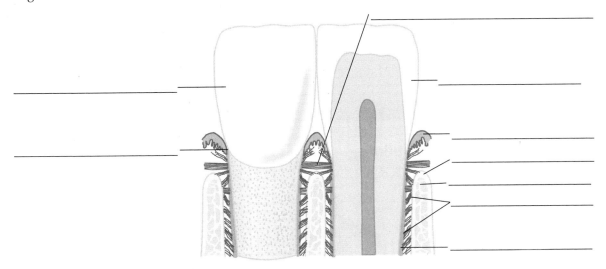

40. Figure 14.32

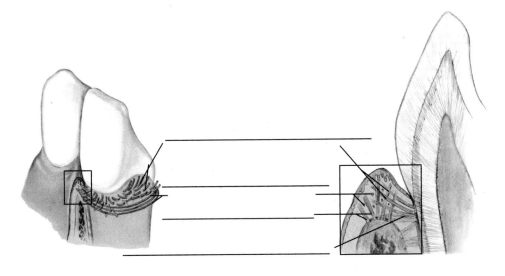

UNIT IV: DENTAL ANATOMY

Chapter 15: Overview of Dentitions

1. Figure 15.1

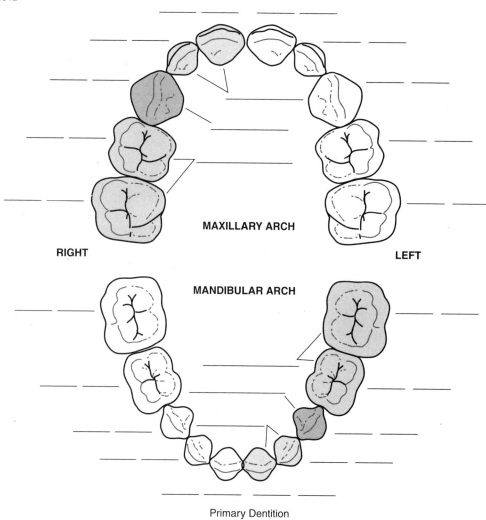

MAXILLARY ARCH

RIGHT   LEFT

MANDIBULAR ARCH

Primary Dentition

2. Figure 15.2

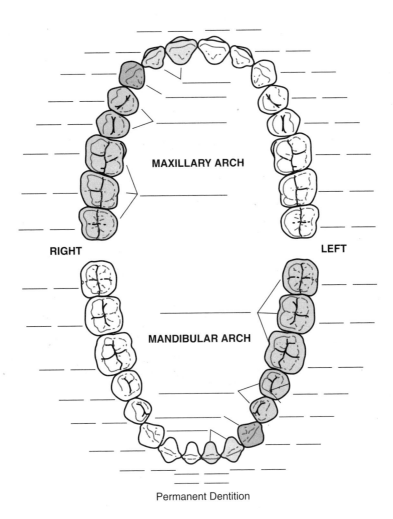

MAXILLARY ARCH

RIGHT   LEFT

MANDIBULAR ARCH

Permanent Dentition

3. Figure 15.5

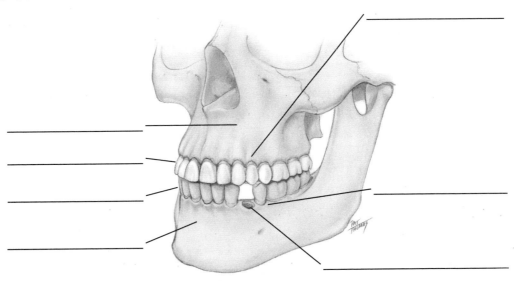

4. Figure 15.6

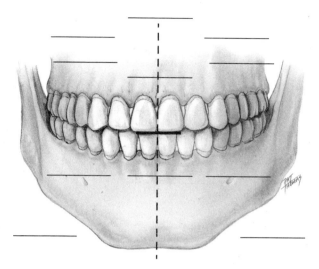

5. Figure 15.7

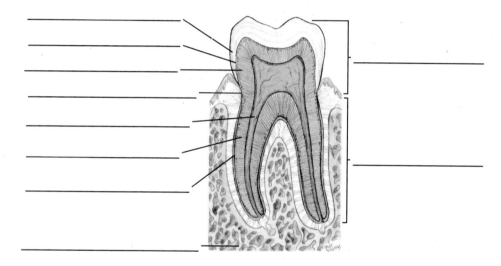

6. Figure 15.8

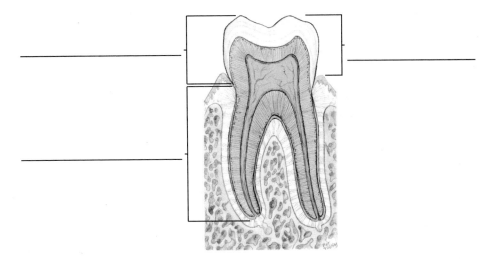

7. Figure 15.9

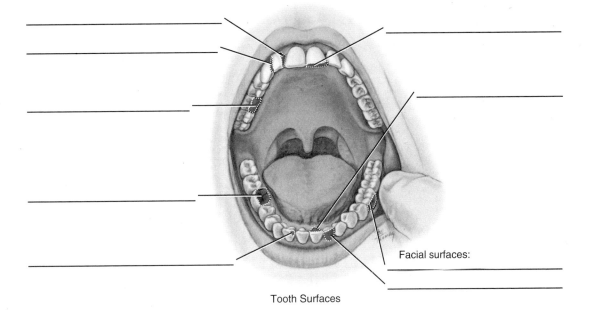

Facial surfaces:

Tooth Surfaces

8. Figure 15.11

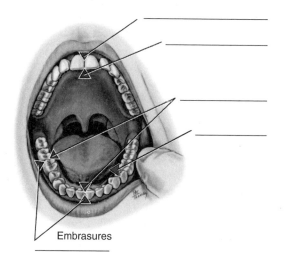

Embrasures

9. Figure 15.12

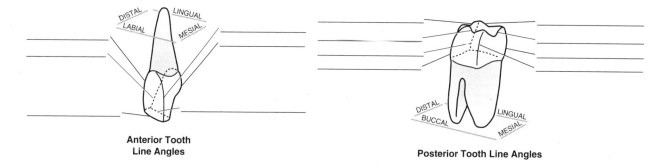

**Anterior Tooth
Line Angles**

Posterior Tooth Line Angles

10. Figure 15.14

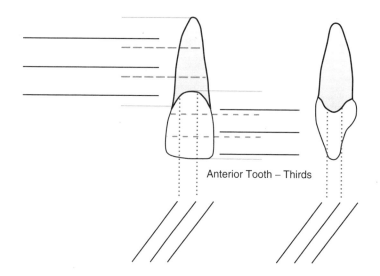

Anterior Tooth – Thirds

11. Figure 15.14 (continued)

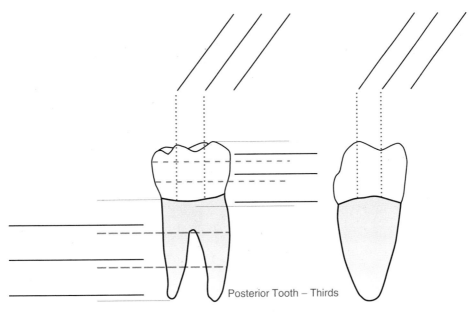

Posterior Tooth – Thirds

Chapter 16: Permanent Anterior Teeth

12. Figure 16.7

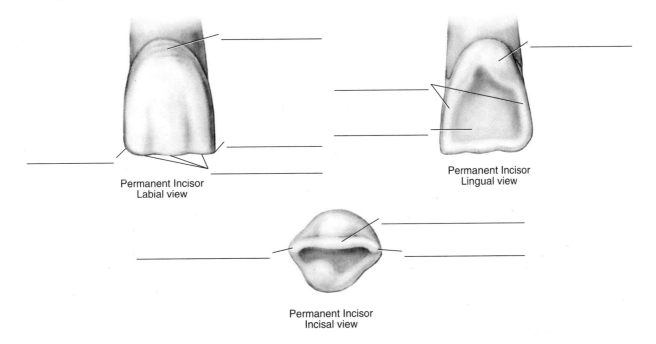

Permanent Incisor
Labial view

Permanent Incisor
Lingual view

Permanent Incisor
Incisal view

13. Figure 16.16

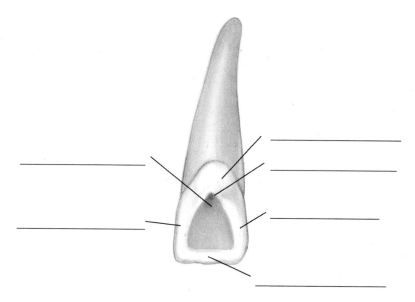

Permanent Maxillary Right Lateral Incisor
Lingual View

14. Figure 16.22

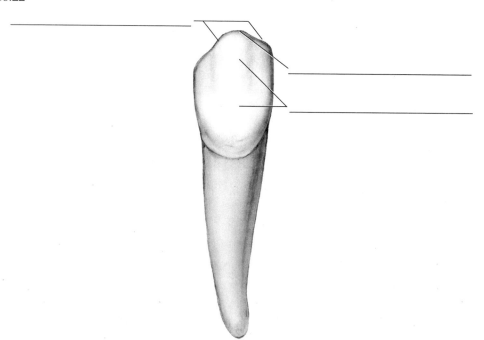

Permanent Mandibular Right Canine
Labial View

15. Figure 16.23

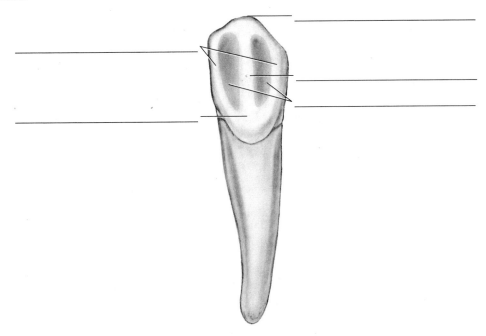

Permanent Mandibular Right Canine
Lingual View

16. Figure 16.27

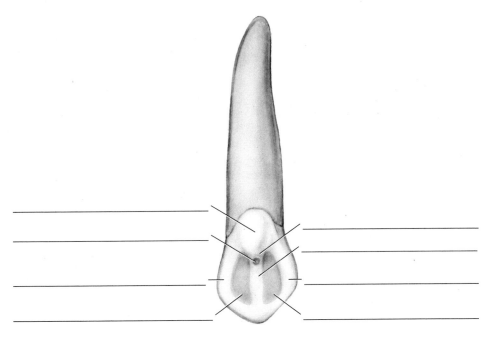

Permanent Maxillary Right Canine
Lingual View

Chapter 17: Permanent Posterior Teeth

17. Figure 17.2

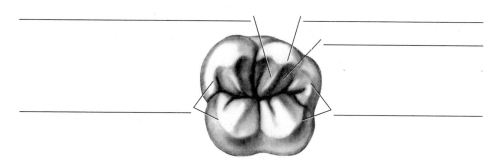

Permanent Posterior Tooth
Occlusal View

18. Figure 17.4

Developmental Grooves:

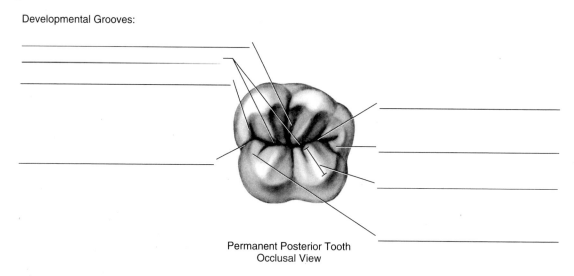

Permanent Posterior Tooth
Occlusal View

19. Figure 17.7

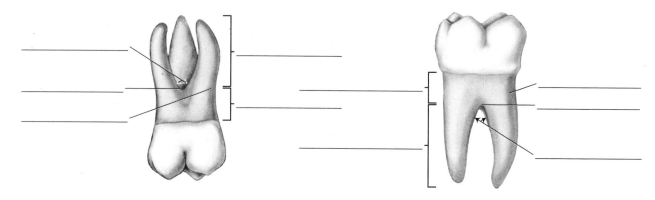

Permanent Posterior Molars: Maxillary and Mandibular
Buccal Views

20. Figure 17.10

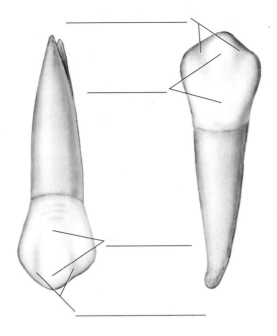

Permanent Premolars
Buccal Views

21. Figure 17.13

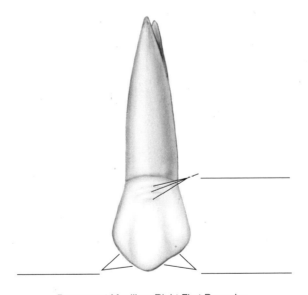

Permanent Maxillary Right First Premolar
Buccal View

22. Figure 17.14, *A, B*

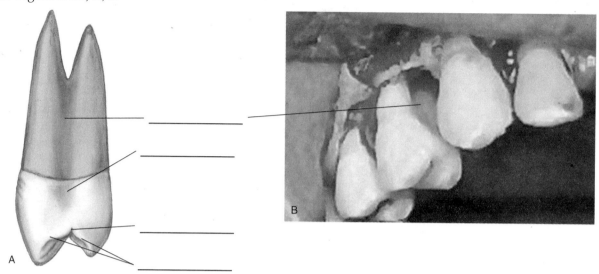

23. Figure 17.15

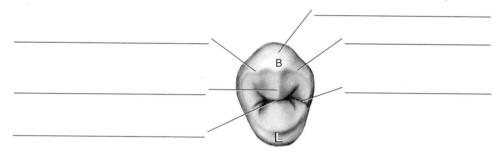

Permanent Maxillary Right First Premolar
Occlusal View

24. Figure 17.16

Transverse {
Ridge {

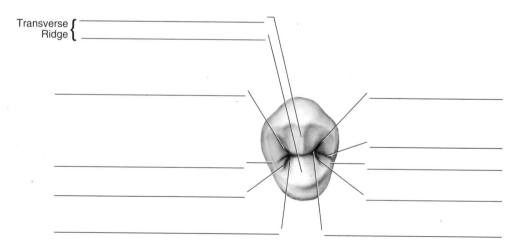

Permanent Maxillary Right First Premolar
Occlusal View

25. Figure 17.19

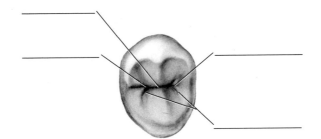

Permanent Maxillary Right Second Premolar
Occlusal View

26. Figure 17.22

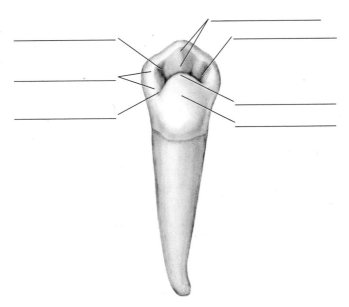

Permanent Mandibular Right First Premolar
Lingual View

27. Figure 17.23

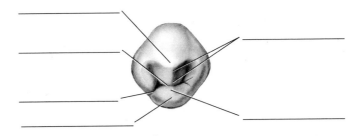

Permanent Mandibular Right First Premolar
Occlusal View

28. Figure 17.24

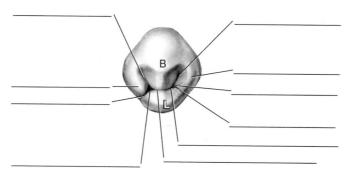

Permanent Mandibular Right First Premolar
Occlusal View

29. Figure 17.27

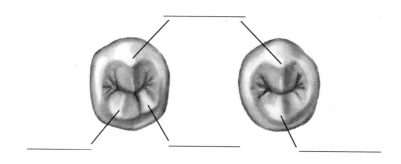

Three-Cusp type   **Two-Cusp type**

Permanent Mandibular Second Premolars
Occlusal Views

30. Figure 17.29

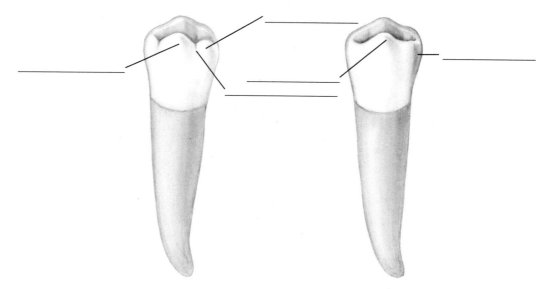

Three-Cusp type   **Two-Cusp type**

Permanent Mandibular Right First Premolars
Lingual Views

31. Figure 17.30

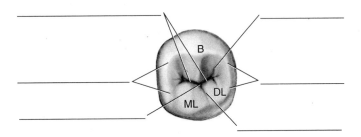

Permanent Mandibular Right Second Premolar: Three-Cusp Type, Y-Shaped Groove Pattern
Occlusal View

32. Figure 17.31

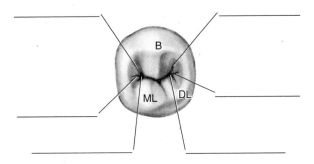

Permanent Mandibular Right Second Premolar: Three-Cusp Type
Occlusal View

33. Figure 17.32

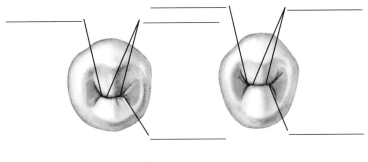

**U-Shaped
Groove Pattern**   **H-Shaped
Groove Pattern**

Permanent Mandibular Right Second Premolars: Two-Cusp Type
Occlusal View

34. Figure 17.34

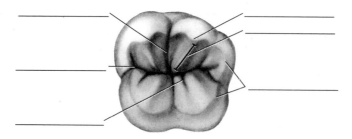

Permanent Molar
Occlusal View

35. Figure 17.37

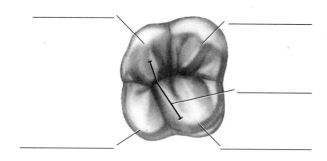

Permanent Maxillary Molar
Occlusal View

36. Figure 17.41

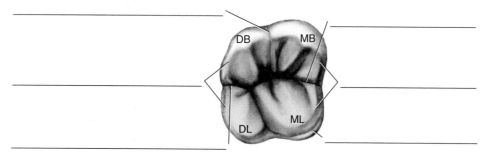

Permanent Maxillary Right First Molar
Occlusal View

37. Figure 17.42

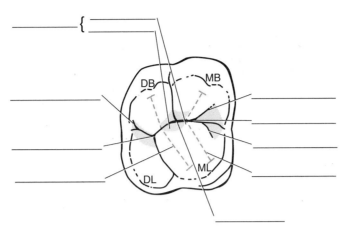

Permanent Maxillary Right First Molar
Occlusal View

38. Figure 17.46

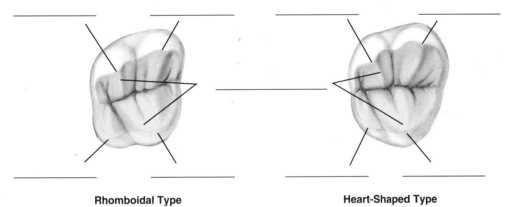

Rhomboidal Type   **Heart-Shaped Type**

Permanent Maxillary Right Second Molars
Occlusal Views

39. Figure 17.53

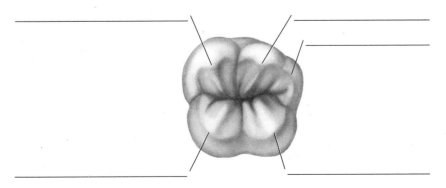

Permanent Mandibular Right First Molar
Occlusal View

40. Figure 17.54

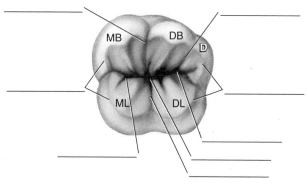

Permanent Maxillary Right First Molar
Occlusal View

41. Figure 17.59

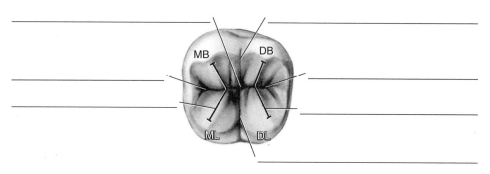

Permanent Mandibular Right Second Molar
Occlusal View

Chapter 18: Primary Dentition

42. Figure 18.2

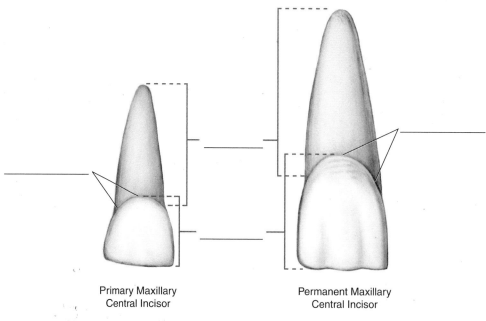

Primary Maxillary
Central Incisor

Permanent Maxillary
Central Incisor

Labial Views

43. Figure 18.3

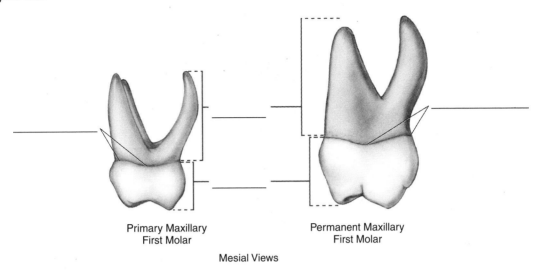

Primary Maxillary
First Molar

Permanent Maxillary
First Molar

Mesial Views

Chapter 19: Temporomandibular Joint

44. Figure 19.1

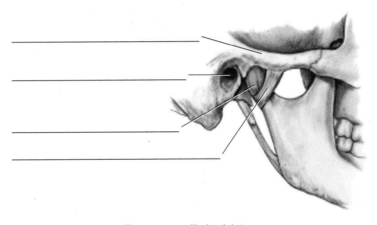

Temporomandibular Joint

45. Figure 19.5

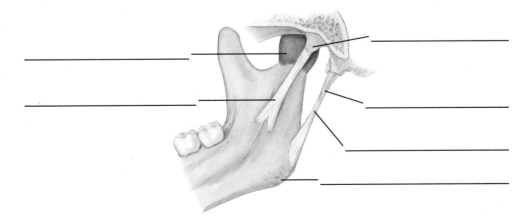

46. Figure 19.6

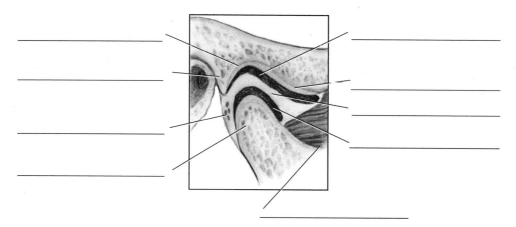

47. Figure 19.8, *A*, *B*, *C*

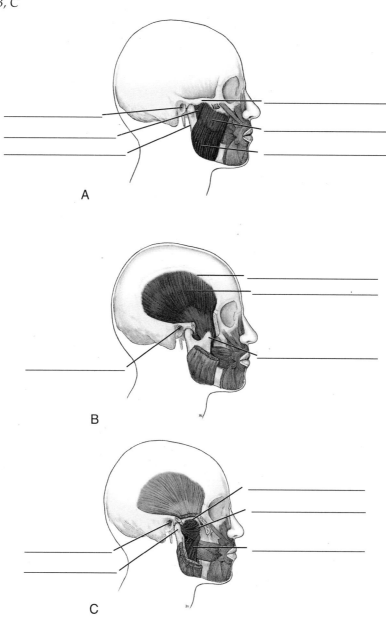

A

B

C

Basic Clinical Supplies Needed: The student dental professional will need the following basic supplies for the clinical identification exercises: dental chair and light, mirror instrument, hand mirror, and workbook-included checklist. Standard infection control precautions, including personal protection equipment, must be adhered to as outlined by the Occupational Safety and Health Administration Bloodborne Pathogens Standard (see reference in Infection Control Procedures for Extracted Teeth). Both Universal and International Numbering Systems are included in the checklists.

After completing the medical and dental history and review, the patient should be seated in a dental chair, either supine or upright as needed. Use preprocedural antimicrobial mouthrinse, remove any pigmented lipsticks, and apply nonpetroleum lubricant to dry lips; ask to take out any removable prostheses. Good lighting and exposure of the area being assessed are essential (e.g., collar and tie loosened, glasses removed).

Explanations of the reasons for performing extraoral and intraoral examinations for the patient as well as examination of the dentition and occlusion and their relationship of these examinations to dental treatment, including the terms used in these examinations, are located in the associated textbook in **Chapters 1, 2, 15, and 20**. More in-depth examination of these areas can be done in the future by student dental professionals after additional coursework in oral pathology, periodontology, dental materials, radiology, and clinical rotations.

Part 1: CLINICAL IDENTIFICATION EXERCISE: Extraoral Structures

Directions: During this exercise in extraoral structure identification, check the items as noted. Use both visual inspection and palpation during the examination, making sure to also note any variations such as with traumatic injury, if applicable. Include specific location using nearby structures. Also note any atypical findings; if found, take nonidentifiable clinical photographs to be shared (after being granted permission) with other students and make appropriate referrals. Include also any palpable lymph nodes of the face and neck, if applicable.

Regions of the Face Checklist		
Frontal, Orbital, and Nasal Regions	**Variations**	**Atypical Findings**
Forehead		
Orbits		
External Nose: Root of Nose, Apex of Nose, Nares, Nasal Septum, Nasal Alae		
Infraorbital and Zygomatic Regions	**Variations**	**Atypical Findings**
Zygomatic Arches		
Temporomandibular Joints		
Buccal Regions	**Variations**	**Atypical Findings**
Cheeks and Masseter Muscles		
Angles of the Mandible		
Parotid Salivary Glands		
Oral Region	**Variations**	**Atypical Findings**
Lips: Vermilion Zones/Borders, Mucocutaneous Junctions, Labial Commissures		
Maxillae, Philtrum, Tubercle of Upper Lip		
Mental Region	**Variations**	**Atypical Findings**
Mandible: Mandibular Symphysis, Rami, Coronoid Processes, Coronoid Notches, Mandibular Condyles, Mandibular Notches		

Regions of the Neck	Variations	Atypical Findings
Sternocleidomastoid Muscles		
Hyoid Bone		
Thyroid Cartilage		
Thyroid Gland		
Submandibular Salivary Glands		
Sublingual Salivary Glands		

Part 2: CLINICAL IDENTIFICATION EXERCISE: Intraoral Structures

Directions: During this exercise in intraoral structure identification, check the items as noted. Use both visual inspection and palpation during the examination, making sure to also note any variations such as Fordyce spots, linea alba, exostoses, mandibular tori, and palatal torus, if applicable. Include specific location using nearby structures. Also note any atypical findings; if found, take nonidentifiable clinical photographs to be shared (after being granted permission) with other students and make appropriate referrals.

The posterior part of the base of the tongue and its structures, such as the lingual tonsil, are usually not visible when examining the oral cavity; however, note the relationship of the nasopharynx and laryngopharynx to the oropharynx by indicating on the external neck the placement of these related internal regions. When examining oral mucosal surfaces, it is important to gently dry those surfaces with a gauze or air syringe, so that color or texture changes will become more obvious. In addition, avoid palpation of any structures near the soft palate or pharynx to prevent the gag reflex; use only visual inspection in this area.

Oral Cavity Checklist		
Oral Vestibules	**Variations**	**Atypical Findings**
Labial Mucosa		
Buccal Mucosa, Buccal Fat Pads		
Parotid Salivary Glands, Parotid Papillae		
Vestibular Fornices		
Alveolar Mucosa, Mucobuccal Folds		
Labial Frena: Maxillary and Mandibular		
Jaws, Alveolar Processes, Teeth, Arches	**Variations**	**Atypical Findings**
Maxillae: Body, Maxillary Sinuses, Alveolar Process, Alveoli, Canine Eminences, Maxillary Teeth, Maxillary Tuberosities		
Mandible: Body, Alveolar Process, Alveoli, Canine Eminences, Mandibular Teeth, Retromolar Pads		
Permanent Teeth within Maxillary and Mandibular Arches: Crowns, Enamel, Anterior Teeth (Incisors, Canines), Posterior Teeth (Premolars, Molars)		

Gingival Tissue	Variations	Atypical Findings
Attached Gingiva		
Mucogingival Junctions		
Marginal Gingiva: Free Gingival Crests and Grooves		
Gingival Sulci (location only)		
Interdental Gingiva: Interdental Papillae		
Oral Cavity Proper	**Variations**	**Atypical Findings**
Fauces: Anterior and Posterior Pillars		
Palatine Tonsils		
Palate	**Variations**	**Atypical Findings**
Hard Palate: Median Palatine Raphe, Incisive Papilla, Palatine Rugae		
Soft Palate, Uvula		
Pterygomandibular Folds		
Tongue	**Variations**	**Atypical Findings**
Base of Tongue (anterior part only)		
Body of Tongue		
Dorsal Surface: Median Lingual Sulcus, Sulcus Terminalis, Foramen Cecum (if possible)		
Filiform Lingual Papillae		
Circumvallate Lingual Papillae		
Lateral Surfaces		
Foliate Lingual Papillae		
Ventral Surface		
Plicae Fimbriatae		
Floor of the Mouth	**Variations**	**Atypical Findings**
Lingual Frenum		
Sublingual Folds		
Sublingual Caruncles		
Sublingual Salivary Glands		
Submandibular Salivary Glands		
Pharynx	**Variations**	**Atypical Findings**
Oropharynx		

Part 3: CLINICAL IDENTIFICATION EXERCISE: Tooth Types in Permanent Dentition

Directions: During this exercise in identifying tooth types in the permanent dentition, circle the items as noted on the crowns of the tooth types listed. Place NA (Not Applicable) if trauma, restoration, or extraction has occurred to the tooth crown so that it is impossible to tell what is present; third molars will not be specifically examined, but take notes on crown anatomy, if present. Compare both sides of each arch when investigating; the sequence below is the same as the one used for discussion in the associated textbook. Use both the instrument mirror and explorer during the examination, making sure to also note any variations or atypical findings; if found, take nonidentifiable clinical photographs to be shared (after being granted permission) with other students and make appropriate referrals.

INCISORS CHECKLIST

TOOTH NUMBER	INCISAL SURFACE	CINGULUM/ MARGINAL RIDGES	LINGUAL FOSSA	NOTES
8, 9 (11, 21)	Ridge/Edge	Well-developed/ Not noticeable	Deep/Shallow	
7, 10 (12, 22)	Ridge/Edge	Well-developed/ Not noticeable	Deep/Shallow	
24, 25 (31, 41)	Ridge/Edge	Well-developed/ Not noticeable	Deep/Shallow	
23, 26 (32, 42)	Ridge/Edge	Well-developed/ Not noticeable	Deep/Shallow	

CANINES CHECKLIST

TOOTH NUMBER	CUSP TIP	CINGULUM/ LINGUAL RIDGE/ MARGINAL RIDGES	LINGUAL FOSSA	NOTES
6, 11 (13, 23)	Centered/ Offset	Well-developed/Not noticeable	Deep/Shallow	
22, 27 (33, 43)	Centered/ Offset	Well-developed/Not noticeable	Deep/Shallow	

PREMOLARS CHECKLIST

TOOTH NUMBER	OCCLUSAL SHAPE	CUSPS	RIDGES	PROXIMAL SHAPE	NOTES
5, 12 (14, 24)	Hexagonal/Diamond-Shaped/Square	2 or 3	Transverse/ Not Transverse	Trapezoidal/ Rhomboidal	
4, 13 (15, 25)	Hexagonal/Diamond-Shaped/Square	2 or 3	Transverse/ Not Transverse	Trapezoidal/ Rhomboidal	
21, 28 (34, 44)	Hexagonal/Diamond-Shaped/Square	2 or 3	Transverse/ Not Transverse	Trapezoidal/ Rhomboidal	
20, 29 (35, 45)	Hexagonal/Diamond-Shaped/Square	2 or 3	Transverse/Not Transverse	Trapezoidal/ Rhomboidal	

MOLARS CHECKLIST

TOOTH NUMBER	OCCLUSAL SHAPE	CUSPS	RIDGES	PROXIMAL SHAPE	PITS	NOTES
3, 14 (16, 26)	Rhomboidal/ Heart-Shaped	4 or 5	Oblique/ Transverse	Trapezoidal/ Rhomboidal	Lingual/ Buccal	
2, 15 (17, 27)	Rhomboidal/ Heart-Shaped	4 or 5	Oblique/ Transverse	Trapezoidal/ Rhomboidal	Lingual/ Buccal	
19, 30 (36, 46)	Rectangular/ Pentagonal	4 or 5	Oblique/ Transverse	Trapezoidal/ Rhomboidal	Lingual/ Buccal	
18, 31 (37, 47)	Rectangular/ Pentagonal	4 or 5	Oblique/ Transverse	Trapezoidal/ Rhomboidal	Lingual/ Buccal	
1, 16 (18, 28)						
17, 32 (38, 48)						

Part 4: CLINICAL IDENTIFICATION EXERCISE: Permanent Dentition Occlusion

Additional Supplies Needed: The student dental professional will need the following additional supplies during these exercises for the clinical identification of an occlusion of a permanent dentition: periodontal probe instrument, articulating paper, and floss. Because many steps are involved in this procedure, the sequence executed can be modified as needed; the following sequence is the same as the one during the related discussion in the associated textbook. If there are interesting features to the occlusion, take nonidentifiable clinical photographs to be shared (after being granted permission) with other students and make appropriate referrals.

Step 1. Occlusal History With Extraoral and Intraoral Findings

Before performing the identification of an occlusion, take notes on the **occlusal history** of the patient. Note in the chart any removable prostheses (flippers, retainers, night and sports mouthguards, and partial or complete dentures), and have the patient keep them in during the procedure if worn regularly. Record any occlusal complaints, habits, and applicable physical or psychological findings from the patient or medical history questionnaire that may be pertinent to the patient's occlusal history. Note these findings under occlusal history.

Additionally, include any additional notes found during an **extraoral examination** that may be pertinent to the patient's occlusion (see earlier discussion). This includes the facial profile, asymmetries, loss of vertical dimension, mandibular deviation upon opening, and temporomandibular disorder signs. Also include any notes found during an intraoral examination that may be pertinent to the patient's occlusion. Note the general amount of **attrition** or **abfraction** of the dentition and record the location and amount of any associated **wear facet** or **cervical lesion** involved in the area provided on the chart. Finally, note any **mobility** of the dentition by circling the involved teeth in red opposite the mobility section.

Record any **sensitivity** to thermal changes or percussion (gentle tapping). Record any deviations in the **intra-arch form or alignment**, such as loss of contact, plunging cusps, open bite, crossbites, and any arch collapse. Note also any missing, rotated, supererupted, drifted, or fractured teeth, as well as those with abfraction. Include any changes in restorations; occlusal trauma is the main reason for early restoration failure. Changes in the midline of the two dentitions should also be noted. Note these items related to intra-arch findings in the areas listed on the chart.

Finally, record any pertinent information from a **radiographic examination** of the dentition, if available, such as amount of bone support, alterations of the periodontal ligament, root resorption, and nonvital and fixed prosthetic teeth, including veneers, crowns, and implants. Record these findings in the area listed as the radiographic examination.

Step 2. Achieving Centric Relation Through Patient–Clinician Positioning

To allow the student dental professional to identify the occlusion of a patient, the patient must be first in **centric relation (CR)**. The position of CR is the end point of closure of the mandible in which the mandible is in the most retruded position, which will serve as a baseline for an occlusal evaluation.

To achieve CR, first place the patient in an upright position, sitting or standing in front and to the side of the patient. The patient should be relaxed, looking straight ahead with lips parted. Using the operating hand, place a thumb against the outside of the patient's chin, with the fingers placed under the inferior border of the mandible to alternately lift and loosen the mandible. Then establish the hinge movement of the mandible by gently arcing the mandible with the fingers several times in a closing and opening manner. Then guide the loosened mandible into closure, with the mandible placed in its most retruded position.

Step 3. Determining Angle Classification of Malocclusion

Once the patient is in CR, determine the **Angle classification of malocclusion** of the patient's dentition. Most cases can be placed into one of three main classes on the basis of the position of the permanent maxillary first molar relative to the mandibular first molar (see text). The position of the canines in each arch must also be noted if the first molars cannot be used for classification. A tendency to any type of malocclusion, which is considered less than the width of a premolar, can be noted using either the molar or canine relationship. Additionally, any subgroups within the classification must be noted as well if the right or left side is not symmetrical in classification. The classification is recorded in the area on the chart labeled "Angle classification."

Step 4. Measuring Overjet

With the patient maintained in CR, **overjet** or horizontal overlap between the two arches is determined by measuring it in millimeters with the tip of the periodontal probe. Place the probe at a right angle to the labial surface of a mandibular incisor at the base of the incisal ridge of a maxillary incisor. The measurement is taken from the labial surface of the mandibular incisor to the lingual surface of the maxillary incisor. Note that the labiolingual width of the maxillary incisor is not included in the measurement. The overjet measurement is recorded in the chart in the area labeled "Overjet."

Step 5. Measuring Overbite

Overbite or vertical overlap between the two arches is determined also by measuring it in millimeters with the tip of the periodontal probe after the patient is placed in CR. Place the probe on the incisal ridge of the maxillary incisor at a right angle to the mandibular incisor. As the patient opens the mouth or depresses the jaws, then place the probe vertically against the mandibular incisor to measure the distance to the incisal ridge of the mandibular incisor. The overbite measurement is recorded in the chart in the area labeled "Overbite."

Step 6. Checking for Interocclusal Clearance

Allow the patient to rest while checking for **interocclusal clearance**, the space when the mandible is at rest. In this rest position, an average space of 2 to 3 mm can be noted between the masticatory surfaces of the maxillary and mandibular teeth. Thus failure of a patient to assume this position when the jaws are not at work may mean the patient is habitually tense or has a **parafunctional habit** such as clenching or grinding (bruxism). Interocclusal clearance is measured in millimeters and recorded in that area on the chart. If there is no interocclusal clearance noted during mandibular rest, follow-up questions may be necessary to ascertain any habitual tension or a parafunctional habit.

Step 7. Checking for Premature Contact

After the patient relaxes for a moment the position of CR can again be attained and the patient is then asked where the teeth first touch during occlusion by having them close their teeth gently together. If it is a single tooth, the tooth is considered to be a premature contact. Articulation paper can then be used to check for any **premature contact**, which limits the opportunity for maximal intercuspation of the teeth. Any premature contact is recorded in the chart by circling the tooth numbers of the contacting teeth in red opposite the CR occlusion section.

Step 8. Achieving Centric Occlusion

Next, have the patient clench the teeth together and note the amount of shift in millimeters from jaw position in CR to jaw position in **centric occlusion (CO)** as well as its direction. CO or habitual occlusion is the voluntary position of the dentition that allows maximal contact when the teeth occlude. Record the amount of shift in millimeters in the chart; record also the direction of the shift (anterior, right, left, posterior). Ideally, no shift is noted because the position of the teeth in CR is the same as in CO; CR = CO is circled in the chart. However, the average distance of shift from a patient's occlusion in CR to CO is approximately 1 mm or less, in an anterior-to-posterior direction.

Step 9. Checking Lateral Occlusion

Next, it is necessary to check the patient's occlusion within lateral deviation or excursion. **Lateral occlusion** is evaluated by moving the mandible to either the right or the left until the canines on that side are in **canine rise** or cuspid rise. The patient's mandible is supported with the operating hand and then the mandible is gently moved into CR or even CO. Then slowly guide the mandible to the patient's right or left until the opposing canines are edge-to-edge.

The side to which the mandible has been moved is the **working side**. There are two working sides noted in an occlusal evaluation: right lateral and left lateral. Before the opposing canines come into contact on each side, other individual teeth that make contact on the working side should be noted. Any **working contact** is recorded by circling the tooth numbers of the contacting teeth in blue on the chart in the area opposite the lateral occlusion section for the appropriate side.

The side of the arch that is opposite or contralateral to the working side during lateral occlusion is the **balancing side** or nonworking side. If any teeth make contact on the balancing side during lateral occlusion, they are recorded as a **balancing interference** and are circled in red for the appropriate side. If group function is present, most of the entire posterior quadrant of each arch is functioning during lateral occlusion without canine rise. This should be recorded by circling the tooth numbers of the involved group of teeth in blue on the chart opposite the lateral occlusion section for the appropriate side.

Do not allow patients to move freely into lateral deviation because they may choose a convenient path to bypass a balancing interference within the occlusion. For further confirmation of any balancing interferences during lateral deviation, place floss across the retromolar pads extending out to the labial commissures or place articulating paper over the occlusal surfaces on the appropriate side. After guiding the patient into either right or left lateral occlusion, slip the floss or articulating paper forward, noting any points of contact.

Step 10. Checking Protrusive Occlusion

Finally, check the **protrusive occlusion** of the patient. With the patient's teeth in CO, support the mandible with the operating hand and have the patient slowly move the mandible forward so that the two dentitions are in an edge-to-edge relationship. Note any posterior tooth or canine contacts as well as any **balancing interference** during protrusion and record this information on the chart by circling the contacting teeth in red opposite the protrusive section. Also note the anterior teeth that are in contact during protrusion or any **working contact** by circling on the chart the tooth numbers of the contacting teeth in blue opposite the protrusive section.

For further confirmation of working contacts and any balancing interferences during protrusion, place the floss across the retromolar pads extending out to the labial commissures. Then guide the patient into protrusive occlusion and slip the floss forward between the teeth until resistance of contacting teeth is met.

OCCLUSAL IDENTIFICATION FORM

Occlusal History _____

Extraoral Findings _____

Intraoral Findings _____

Angle Classification _____ Right _____ Left _____ Subgroup _____

Molar Right _____ Canine Right _____ Molar Left _____ Canine Left _____

Interocclusal Clearance _____ mm   Sensitivity _____

Overjet ____ mm   Overbite ____ mm

Attrition _____ Abfraction _____

Intra-Arch Form/Alignment _____

Radiographic Examination (if available) _____

OCCLUSAL IDENTIFICATION CHECKLIST

Centric Relation **Centric Occlusion**	1 (18	2 17	3 16	4 15	5 14	6 13	7 12	8 11)	9 (21	10 22	11 23	12 24	13 25	14 26	15 27	16 28)
	32 (48	31 47	30 46	29 45	28 44	27 43	26 42	25 41)	24 (31	23 32	22 33	21 34	20 35	19 36	18 37	17 38)
CR = CO	Shift CR to CO ____ mm								Anterior Right Left Posterior							
Right Lateral **Occlusion**	1 (18	2 17	3 16	4 15	5 14	6 13	7 12	8 11)	9 (21	10 22	11 23	12 24	13 25	14 26	15 27	16 28)
	32 (48	31 47	30 46	29 45	28 44	27 43	26 42	25 41)	24 (31	23 32	22 33	21 34	20 35	19 36	18 37	17 38)
Left Lateral **Occlusion**	1 (18	2 17	3 16	4 15	5 14	6 13	7 12	8 11)	9 (21	10 22	11 23	12 24	13 25	14 26	15 27	16 28)
	32 (48	31 47	30 46	29 45	28 44	27 43	26 42	25 41)	24 (31	23 32	22 33	21 34	20 35	19 36	18 37	17 38)
Protrusive **Occlusion**	1 (18	2 17	3 16	4 15	5 14	6 13	7 12	8 11)	9 (21	10 22	11 23	12 24	13 25	14 26	15 27	16 28)
	32 (48	31 47	30 46	29 45	28 44	27 43	26 42	25 41)	24 (31	23 32	22 33	21 34	20 35	19 36	18 37	17 38)
Wear Facet	1 (18	2 17	3 16	4 15	5 14	6 13	7 12	8 11)	9 (21	10 22	11 23	12 24	13 25	14 26	15 27	16 28)
	32 (48	31 47	30 46	29 45	28 44	27 43	26 42	25 41)	24 (31	23 32	22 33	21 34	20 35	19 36	18 37	17 38)
Cervical Lesion	1 (18	2 17	3 16	4 15	5 14	6 13	7 12	8 11)	9 (21	10 22	11 23	12 24	13 25	14 26	15 27	16 28)
	32 (48	31 47	30 46	29 45	28 44	27 43	26 42	25 41)	24 (31	23 32	22 33	21 34	20 35	19 36	18 37	17 38)
Mobility	1 (18	2 17	3 16	4 15	5 14	6 13	7 12	8 11)	9 (21	10 22	11 23	12 24	13 25	14 26	15 27	16 28)
	32 (48	31 47	30 46	29 45	28 44	27 43	26 42	25 41)	24 (31	23 32	22 33	21 34	20 35	19 36	18 37	17 38)

PART 1: CHAPTER WORD JUMBLES

Note: Answers can be obtained from your instructor and their Evolve Resources

Chapter 1: Face and Neck Regions

1. *Lower jaw* LEDIBMAN ☐☐☐☐☐☐☐☐
2. *Ramus part* ONORIDCO ☐☐☐☐☐☐☐☐
3. *Kisser corner* SUREMISCOM ☐☐☐☐☐☐☐☐☐☐
4. *Muscle mania* TERSEMAS ☐☐☐☐☐☐☐☐
5. *In thyroid* DOIRTHYARAP ☐☐☐☐☐☐☐☐☐☐☐
6. *Cheeky gland* TIDROPA ☐☐☐☐☐☐☐
7. *Upper lip thick* UERBCLET ☐☐☐☐☐☐☐☐
8. *Upper lip dip* TURIMLPH ☐☐☐☐☐☐☐☐
9. *Head joint* MANBTOROPDIULAREM ☐☐☐☐☐☐☐☐☐☐☐☐☐☐☐☐☐
10. *Lipstick home* LIONMIREV ☐☐☐☐☐☐☐☐☐

Chapter 2: Oral Cavity and Pharynx

1. *Misplaced oil* ODRCYEF ☐☐☐☐☐☐☐
2. *Dog teeth* NESNICA ☐☐☐☐☐☐☐
3. *Grinding fun* CASTIMIOATN ☐☐☐☐☐☐☐☐☐☐☐
4. *Arch bumps* SESXTOESO ☐☐☐☐☐☐☐☐☐
5. *Tooth padding* VAINGGI ☐☐☐☐☐☐☐
6. *Entrance walls* UFALAIC ☐☐☐☐☐☐☐
7. *Tongue specials* LALAPPIE ☐☐☐☐☐☐☐☐
8. *Tongue line-up* VALARICTMUCE ☐☐☐☐☐☐☐☐☐☐☐☐
9. *Bony arches* EORVALAL ☐☐☐☐☐☐☐☐
10. *Mushroom-shape specials* GORMFUNIF ☐☐☐☐☐☐☐☐☐

Chapter 3: Prenatal Development

1. *Cavity fluid* TICNAIMO ☐☐☐☐☐☐☐

2. *Outer skin layer* MEERCODT ☐☐☐☐☐☐☐☐

3. *First divisions* GEAVECLA ☐☐☐☐☐☐☐☐

4. *Genetic map* YOKAPRETY ☐☐☐☐☐☐☐☐☐

5. *Future embryo* TOYSCBALST ☐☐☐☐☐☐☐☐☐☐

6. *Union result* GOTEYZ ☐☐☐☐☐☐

7. *From ectoderm* NETUCREDMOORE ☐☐☐☐☐☐☐☐☐☐☐☐☐

8. *Embryonic tissue* CESHEMENYM ☐☐☐☐☐☐☐☐☐☐

9. *First draft* RORPUDMIMI ☐☐☐☐☐☐☐☐☐☐

10. *Toxic types* EGRAOENTTS ☐☐☐☐☐☐☐☐☐☐

Chapter 4: Face and Neck Development

1. *Nose bump* RACTIEGAL ☐☐☐☐☐☐☐☐

2. *Gill time* CHIALRANB ☐☐☐☐☐☐☐☐☐

3. *Disappearance act* KEECLM ☐☐☐☐☐☐

4. *Neck bone* DIHOY ☐☐☐☐☐

5. *Sense button* DLAPSECO ☐☐☐☐☐☐☐☐

6. *Outer doughnut part* RATELLA ☐☐☐☐☐☐☐

7. *Opening gives communication* NEEMBARM ☐☐☐☐☐☐☐☐

8. *Four evaginations* CPHOSUE ☐☐☐☐☐☐☐

9. *Upper facial place* SOOFNTNAARL ☐☐☐☐☐☐☐☐☐☐☐

10. *Primitive oral landmark* MTOODEMUS ☐☐☐☐☐☐☐☐☐

Chapter 5: Orofacial Development

1. *Tight tongue* AAGYOINSSKLOL ☐☐☐☐☐☐☐☐☐☐☐☐☐

2. *Parting palate* LETCF ☐☐☐☐☐

3. *From fourth swelling* TEIPLIGOCT ☐☐☐☐☐☐☐☐☐☐

4. *Stacked six* IESGLWLNS ☐☐☐☐☐☐☐☐☐

5. *Funny throat thing* AULVU ☐☐☐☐☐

6. *Overgrowing base* OUPALC ☐☐☐☐☐☐

7. *Middle meeting* LESVHSE ☐☐☐☐☐☐☐

8. *Roof parts* AALPLAT ☐☐☐☐☐☐☐

9. *Initial tongue blob* RETMCUBUUL ☐☐☐☐☐☐☐☐☐☐

10. *In midline* AIPRM ☐☐☐☐☐

Chapter 6: Tooth Development and Eruption

1. *Empty slot* OOAANDINT ☐☐☐☐☐☐☐☐☐

2. *Leftover cells* ZELSMAAS ☐☐☐☐☐☐☐☐

3. *Twining trouble* NOIEGMIATN ☐☐☐☐☐☐☐☐☐☐

4. *Primary shedders* STOSLAODNTOC ☐☐☐☐☐☐☐☐☐☐☐☐

5. *Early bony-like form* IOMCEETND ☐☐☐☐☐☐☐☐☐

6. *Secretory surface* SMTEO ☐☐☐☐☐

7. *Compressed layer* MMDIUNTREEI ☐☐☐☐☐☐☐☐☐☐☐

8. *Second draft* NUUCDSCEAEOS ☐☐☐☐☐☐☐☐☐☐☐☐

9. *Merry myth* YIFAR ☐☐☐☐☐

10. *Accessory cusps* BEECLSTUR ☐☐☐☐☐☐☐☐☐

Chapter 7: Cells

1. *Cytoplasm spaces* VAUCLEOS ☐☐☐☐☐☐☐☐

2. *Splitting up* SOMTIIS ☐☐☐☐☐☐☐

3. *Junction tie* DOSMMEOSE ☐☐☐☐☐☐☐☐☐

4. *Cell center* ULCELOUNS ☐☐☐☐☐☐☐☐☐

5. *Moving out* OSSEYTOXIC ☐☐☐☐☐☐☐☐☐☐

6. *Breaking down* MESYSLOOS ☐☐☐☐☐☐☐☐☐

7. *Chromatin condenses* ROSHAEPP ☐☐☐☐☐☐☐☐

8. *Two chromatids* TEMRONEECR ☐☐☐☐☐☐☐☐☐☐

9. *Rough guys* SRIMBOOES ☐☐☐☐☐☐☐☐☐

10. *Major player* FEMSTOINNOLAT ☐☐☐☐☐☐☐☐☐☐☐☐☐

Chapter 8: Basic Tissue

1. *Mineral identification* PAAYTHRIODXYTE ☐☐☐☐☐☐☐☐☐☐☐☐
2. *Nutrition canals* CIALNAULIC ☐☐☐☐☐☐☐☐☐
3. *Vessel wrapping* THELENDOMUI ☐☐☐☐☐☐☐☐☐☐☐
4. *Layered epithelium* EFADISTRTI ☐☐☐☐☐☐☐☐☐
5. *Hard rings* TONESSO ☐☐☐☐☐☐☐
6. *Making fibers* BIABSLFROT ☐☐☐☐☐☐☐☐☐
7. *Alien stuff* NIOMUMENG ☐☐☐☐☐☐☐☐
8. *Replacement clocking* ORVENTUR ☐☐☐☐☐☐☐☐
9. *Clot creation* TELLEPAST ☐☐☐☐☐☐☐☐
10. *Nerve communication* NYSASEP ☐☐☐☐☐☐☐

Chapter 9: Oral Mucosa

1. *Unique tissue* TEZEKPAIRNADAIR ☐☐☐☐☐☐☐☐☐☐☐☐☐☐
2. *Waterproofing tactic* RAKTENI ☐☐☐☐☐☐☐
3. *Dark spots* LUGREANS ☐☐☐☐☐☐☐☐
4. *Gum tufting* TIGPIPSLN ☐☐☐☐☐☐☐☐
5. *Blood group* ACALPRILY ☐☐☐☐☐☐☐☐
6. *Down deeper* BOSSAMUUC ☐☐☐☐☐☐☐☐
7. *Italy map* PHIRGAEOCG ☐☐☐☐☐☐☐☐☐
8. *Membrane with bony down under* SMUMEPOCEIROTU ☐☐☐☐☐☐☐☐☐☐☐☐☐☐
9. *Tongue field* ZISPAEECLID ☐☐☐☐☐☐☐☐☐☐
10. *Dried up* KEPICRL ☐☐☐☐☐☐☐

Chapter 10: Gingival and Dentogingival Junctional Tissue

1. *Between layers* NALAMI ☐☐☐☐☐☐
2. *Facing tooth* LAVDENINGTOGI ☐☐☐☐☐☐☐☐☐☐☐☐☐
3. *Always young* JOUCTIANNL ☐☐☐☐☐☐☐☐☐
4. *Periodontal playground* LUULSCRA ☐☐☐☐☐☐☐☐

5. *Future fluid measurement* VUCRRIECLA ☐☐☐☐☐☐☐☐☐☐

6. *Growing gums* HYSAPARLEPI ☐☐☐☐☐☐☐☐☐☐☐

7. *Longer teeth* CORSEESIN ☐☐☐☐☐☐☐☐☐

8. *Sore gums* TIINVSGIGI ☐☐☐☐☐☐☐☐☐☐

9. *Deeper disease* KEOPCT ☐☐☐☐☐☐

10. *Continued infection* DIREPOONTIITS ☐☐☐☐☐☐☐☐☐☐☐☐☐

Chapter 11: Head and Neck Structures

1. *Group secretion* SANCIU ☐☐☐☐☐☐

2. *Gland masses* ELFSOLILC ☐☐☐☐☐☐☐☐☐

3. *Node depression* HUISL ☐☐☐☐☐

4. *Bigger grapes* PYHMDAPELONTYAH ☐☐☐☐☐☐☐☐☐☐☐☐☐☐☐

5. *Nasal projections* OCCHENA ☐☐☐☐☐☐☐

6. *Desert place* XOOERASMTI ☐☐☐☐☐☐☐☐☐☐

7. *Head spaces* RANSPALAA ☐☐☐☐☐☐☐☐☐

8. *Damp kisser* ILASAV ☐☐☐☐☐☐

9. *Making thyroxine* DOLICLO ☐☐☐☐☐☐☐

10. *Lymphoid masses* TALOLNSIR ☐☐☐☐☐☐☐☐☐

Chapter 12: Enamel

1. *Breaking crystals* FABTCANRIO ☐☐☐☐☐☐☐☐☐☐

2. *Dark brushes* FUSTT ☐☐☐☐☐

3. *Rubbed out* BANRAISO ☐☐☐☐☐☐☐☐

4. *Faulty enamel* PDSSYILAA ☐☐☐☐☐☐☐☐☐

5. *Short tubules* NIESDSPL ☐☐☐☐☐☐☐☐

6. *Named layers* TRIESZU ☐☐☐☐☐☐☐

7. *Hard rock bands* AICTMBRINIO ☐☐☐☐☐☐☐☐☐☐☐

8. *Worn jewel* NOTATRITI ☐☐☐☐☐☐☐☐☐

9. *Between enamel units* DORNITER ☐☐☐☐☐☐☐☐

10. *Outer getting the groovy on* KYMPERATIA ☐☐☐☐☐☐☐☐☐☐

Chapter 13: Dentin and Pulp

1. *Whole hole* MONFRAE ☐☐☐☐☐☐☐
2. *Disturbed appositional growth* TURCONO ☐☐☐☐☐☐☐
3. *Around middle* CUCPIRAUMPLL ☐☐☐☐☐☐☐☐☐☐☐
4. *First covering* NETMAL ☐☐☐☐☐☐
5. *Around tubes* BUTLERAPIUR ☐☐☐☐☐☐☐☐☐☐☐
6. *Tubule type* TNADELIN ☐☐☐☐☐☐☐☐
7. *Lateral complications* RAOSCECSY ☐☐☐☐☐☐☐☐☐
8. *Avoid ice* VEISHYPIERSNITTY ☐☐☐☐☐☐☐☐☐☐☐☐☐☐☐☐
9. *Named layers* BERNE ☐☐☐☐☐
10. *Inner pain* TULSPIPI ☐☐☐☐☐☐☐☐

Chapter 14: Periodontium: Cementum, Alveolar Process, and Periodontal Ligament

1. *Trouble scaling* PURSS ☐☐☐☐☐
2. *No cells* RACELALUL ☐☐☐☐☐☐☐☐☐
3. *Two kinds* NELMSECTICE ☐☐☐☐☐☐☐☐☐☐☐
4. *Dental nightmare* EUSUDENTOL ☐☐☐☐☐☐☐☐☐☐
5. *Bulk fibers* QUOIBLE ☐☐☐☐☐☐☐
6. *An extra extra* ISHTYMERCEPENSO ☐☐☐☐☐☐☐☐☐☐☐☐☐☐☐
7. *Probing junction* MEECLEMENTONA ☐☐☐☐☐☐☐☐☐☐☐☐☐
8. *Between roots* RACDILTERIUARN ☐☐☐☐☐☐☐☐☐☐☐☐☐☐
9. *Supporting team* TERIMOODPINU ☐☐☐☐☐☐☐☐☐☐☐☐
10. *Ninety degrees* YESHARP ☐☐☐☐☐☐☐

Chapter 15: Overview of Dentitions

1. *Meeting place* TACONCT ☐☐☐☐☐☐☐
2. *Floss heaven/hell* INOXTMERPRIAL ☐☐☐☐☐☐☐☐☐☐☐☐☐
3. *Bite me* SOONCLUIC ☐☐☐☐☐☐☐☐☐
4. *Ortho charting* LEPARM ☐☐☐☐☐☐

5. *Four squares* DANQTUARNS ☐☐☐☐☐☐☐☐☐☐

6. *Linear elevations* GRISED ☐☐☐☐☐☐

7. *Root caves* VITANESCOCI ☐☐☐☐☐☐☐☐☐☐☐

8. *Six slices* XSASENTT ☐☐☐☐☐☐☐☐

9. *More specific* HIRSTD ☐☐☐☐☐☐

10. *Talking points* AUSLNIVER ☐☐☐☐☐☐☐☐☐

Chapter 16: Permanent Anterior Teeth

1. *Traumatic injury* NALVUISO ☐☐☐☐☐☐☐☐

2. *Backside major* CUIMGLUN ☐☐☐☐☐☐☐☐

3. *Older dog tooth term* DUCSPI ☐☐☐☐☐☐

4. *Cute space* STIEAMAD ☐☐☐☐☐☐☐☐

5. *Odd incisor* CHONTUSHIN ☐☐☐☐☐☐☐☐☐☐

6. *Getting depressed* SOAFSE ☐☐☐☐☐☐

7. *Canine retained* PIAMDCET ☐☐☐☐☐☐☐☐

8. *New ridge* SIACLIN ☐☐☐☐☐☐☐

9. *Even cuter* LOESMNAM ☐☐☐☐☐☐☐☐

10. *Extra something* EOSEDIMNS ☐☐☐☐☐☐☐☐☐

Chapter 17: Permanent Posterior Teeth

1. *Older molar friend tag* SPUDICIB ☐☐☐☐☐☐☐☐

2. *Maxillary special* QOEUBIL ☐☐☐☐☐☐☐

3. *Cute cusp* CLERIABAL ☐☐☐☐☐☐☐☐☐

4. *Angular distortion* LEDIARTOCAIN ☐☐☐☐☐☐☐☐☐☐☐☐

5. *Elongated depression* TULFGINT ☐☐☐☐☐☐☐☐

6. *Hidden areas* SHERCOTC ☐☐☐☐☐☐☐☐

7. *Odd molar* BUMLYRER ☐☐☐☐☐☐☐☐

8. *Outside deep groove* UFINSO ☐☐☐☐☐☐

9. *Between roots* AURCFINOT ☐☐☐☐☐☐☐☐☐

10. *Three roots* TERICFRATUD ☐☐☐☐☐☐☐☐☐☐☐

Chapter 18: Primary Dentition

1. *Baby spaces* MIPERAT ⬜⬜⬜⬜⬜⬜⬜
2. *Prominent ridge* RIAVCECL ⬜⬜⬜⬜⬜⬜⬜⬜
3. *Large chamber* LUPP ⬜⬜⬜⬜
4. *Risky restorative moment* NORSH ⬜⬜⬜⬜⬜
5. *Early childhood* SECAIR ⬜⬜⬜⬜⬜⬜
6. *Stained teeth* NAMTHYS ⬜⬜⬜⬜⬜⬜⬜
7. *Good start teeth* MRIYPAR ⬜⬜⬜⬜⬜⬜⬜
8. *Kid grinding* XIRSBUM ⬜⬜⬜⬜⬜⬜⬜
9. *Worn tops* OARNTTITI ⬜⬜⬜⬜⬜⬜⬜⬜⬜
10. *Whiter baby smile* EELANM ⬜⬜⬜⬜⬜⬜

Chapter 19: Temporomandibular Joint

1. *Raising mandible* VEAOINLET ⬜⬜⬜⬜⬜⬜⬜⬜⬜
2. *Inferior depression* CAARITLUR ⬜⬜⬜⬜⬜⬜⬜⬜⬜
3. *Joint fluid* YNOILVSA ⬜⬜⬜⬜⬜⬜⬜⬜
4. *Side movement* TELLARA ⬜⬜⬜⬜⬜⬜⬜
5. *Working muscles* MOICTASAITN ⬜⬜⬜⬜⬜⬜⬜⬜⬜⬜⬜
6. *Sharper ridge* GLOPOSTEDIN ⬜⬜⬜⬜⬜⬜⬜⬜⬜⬜⬜
7. *Partial dislocation* BUIULXATSON ⬜⬜⬜⬜⬜⬜⬜⬜⬜⬜⬜
8. *Joint change* SRIDDORE ⬜⬜⬜⬜⬜⬜⬜⬜
9. *Joint cover* LEAPSCU ⬜⬜⬜⬜⬜⬜⬜
10. *Jaw backward* TROINRACTE ⬜⬜⬜⬜⬜⬜⬜⬜⬜⬜

Chapter 20: Occlusion

1. *Noisy occlusion* MRUIBXS ☐☐☐☐☐☐☐
2. *Mandible facial* TROSBSICE ☐☐☐☐☐☐☐☐☐
3. *Lateral curve* NOLSIW ☐☐☐☐☐☐
4. *Resting mandible* RLEANECAC ☐☐☐☐☐☐☐☐☐
5. *Space for kids* WEEYLA ☐☐☐☐☐☐
6. *Major disharmony* MRATAU ☐☐☐☐☐☐
7. *Habitually centric* OINCUCLSO ☐☐☐☐☐☐☐☐☐
8. *More women* ROIVEEBT ☐☐☐☐☐☐☐
9. *Horizontal overhang* JOEVETR ☐☐☐☐☐☐☐
10. *Occlusal classification* GALNE ☐☐☐☐☐

PART 2: UNIT CROSSWORD PUZZLES

Note: Answers can be obtained from your Instructor and their Evolve Resources

UNIT I: OROFACIAL STRUCTURES

Crossword Puzzle 1

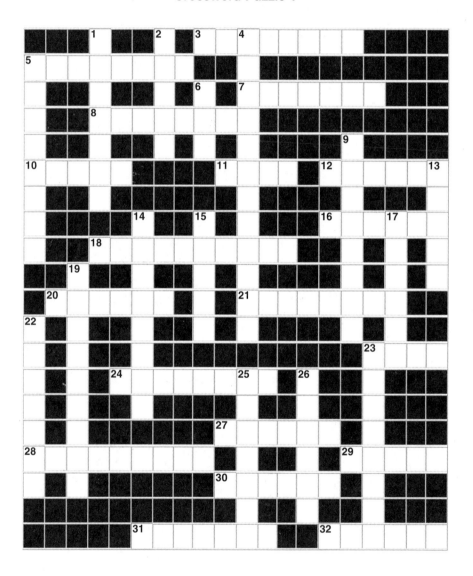

Across

3. Vertical groove noted on midline of upper lip
5. Bony process at anterior border of mandibular ramus
7. Small yellowish oral mucosal elevations from misplaced sebaceous glands
8. Part of maxillae or mandible that supports teeth
10. Nostrils of nose
11. External main feature of nasal region so do not blow it!
12. Structures or facial surfaces of the tooth closest to inner cheek
16. Alveolar process between two neighboring teeth; also called *interdental*
18. Part of the face that contains the lips and oral cavity
20. Hard inner crown layer of tooth overlying pulp
21. Socket of tooth
23. White ridge of raised keratinized epithelial tissue on buccal mucosa
24. Lower jaw
27. Hard outer crown layer of tooth
28. Variation in bone growth on facial surface of maxillary alveolar process
29. Skull socket that contains eyeball and supporting structures
30. Space facing the sulcular epithelium
31. Bony projection off posterior and superior border of mandibular ramus
32. Voice box in midline of neck that is composed of cartilages

Down

1. Opening from the pulp at apex of the tooth
2. Keratinization on inner cheek where the teeth occlude
4. Facial region located both inferior to orbital region and lateral to nasal region
5. Outermost layer of the root of tooth
6. Winglike cartilaginous structure laterally around each nares
9. Midline thickening of the upper lip
13. Tissue fluid that drains from surrounding region into lymphatic vessels
14. Small elevated structures of specialized mucosa on the tongue
15. Depression located where sulcus terminalis points backward toward pharynx
17. Nonencapsulated mass of lymphoid tissue
19. Darker appearance or zone of the lips compared with surrounding skin
22. Anteriors that are also the third teeth from the midline in each quadrant
23. Teeth type that includes incisors and canines located at the front of oral cavity
25. Describes structures or tooth surfaces closest to the tongue
26. Midline tissue fold between ventral surface of the tongue and floor of the mouth

UNIT II: DENTAL EMBRYOLOGY

Crossword Puzzle 1

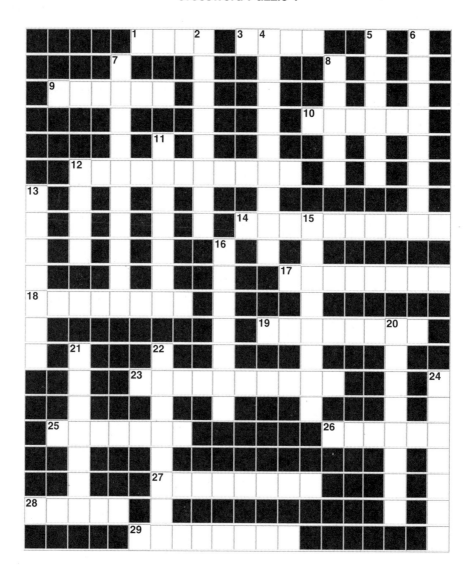

Across

1. Circular plate of bilayered cells developed from blastocyst

3. Depressions in center of each nasal placode that evolve into nasal cavities

9. Elimination of this structure between two adjacent swellings during surface fusion

10. Type of tube formed when neural folds meet and fuse superior to neural groove

12. Cells that differentiate from preameloblasts forming enamel during amelogenesis

14. Overall form of a structure that can undergo change during development

17. Embryonic layer located between ectoderm and endoderm

18. Superior layer of bilaminar embryonic disc

19. Areas of ectoderm found located at developing special sense organs or teeth on embryo

23. Embryonic disc that includes ectoderm, mesoderm, and endoderm

25. Intermaxillary growth from paired medial nasal processes on internal stomodeum

26. Tail end of a structure such as with trilaminar embryonic disc

27. Each half of it mirrors the other half of the embryo because of primitive streak development

28. Structure of fetal period of prenatal development derived from enlarged embryo

29. Process during prenatal development when mitosis converts zygote to blastocyst

Down

2. Head end of structure such as with the trilaminar embryonic disc

4. Action of one cell group on another leading to establishment of developmental pathway

5. Structure derived from implanted blastocyst

6. Posterior one develops from fourth branchial or pharyngeal arches marking future epiglottis

7. Developmental problems evident at birth

8. Specialized cells that develop from neuroectoderm that migrate from neural folds

11. Paired cuboidal aggregates of cells differentiated from the mesoderm

12. Branchial or pharyngeal apparatus part that includes these as well as grooves, membranes, and pouches

13. Cleft lip is fusion failure of maxillary one with medial nasal one on each side

15. Processes that occur from start of pregnancy to birth

16. Membrane at the caudal end of embryo that is the future anus

20. Trilaminar embryonic disc layer derived from epiblast layer that lines stomodeum

21. Anterior part of future digestive tract or primitive pharynx forming oropharynx

22. Membrane that disintegrates bringing nasal and oral cavities into communication

24. Process occurring to embryo that places each embryologic tissue in proper position

UNIT II: DENTAL EMBRYOLOGY

Crossword Puzzle 2

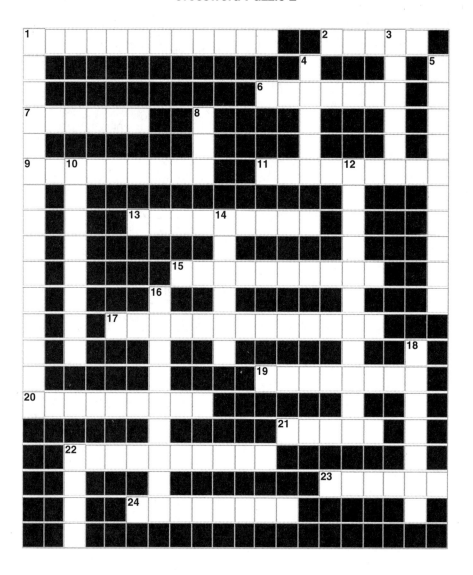

Across

1. Canals that persist after development

2. Fusion failure of palatal shelves with the primary palate or with each other

6. Two palatal processes from maxillary processes during prenatal development

7. Part of cervical loop that shape root or roots inducing root dentin formation

9. Cementum matrix laid down by cementoblasts

11. Circular plate of bilayered cells developed from blastocyst

13. One cell group action that leads to developmental pathway in responding tissue

15. Layered formation of tissue such as cartilage, bone, enamel, dentin, or cementum

17. Process by which sperm penetrates the ovum during preimplantation period

19. Photographic analysis of chromosomes

20. Primitive mouth appearing as shallow depression in embryonic surface

21. Cap or bell-shaped part of tooth germ that produces enamel

22. Prenatal structure of trophoblast cells and inner cell mass that develops into embryo

23. Substance that is partially calcified and serves as framework for later calcification

24. Layer in trilaminar embryonic disc derived from hypoblast layer

Down

1. Permanent teeth type without primary predecessors; also concerns the *molars*

3. Dental developmental disturbance in which adjacent tooth germs unite

4. Small spherical enamel projection near cementoenamel junction

5. Cellular removal of hard tissue such as bone, enamel, dentin, or cementum

8. Second stage of tooth development with dental lamina growth into ectomesenchyme

10. Groups of epithelial cells in periodontal ligament after disintegration of sheath

12. Abnormally small teeth

14. Posterior swellings from third and fourth branchial or pharyngeal arches that overgrow second branchial or pharyngeal arches

16. Dentin matrix laid down through appositional growth by the odontoblasts

18. Process of reproductive cell production that ensures correct number of chromosomes

22. Fourth stage of odontogenesis in which differentiation occurs to its furthest extent

UNIT III: DENTAL HISTOLOGY

Crossword Puzzle 1

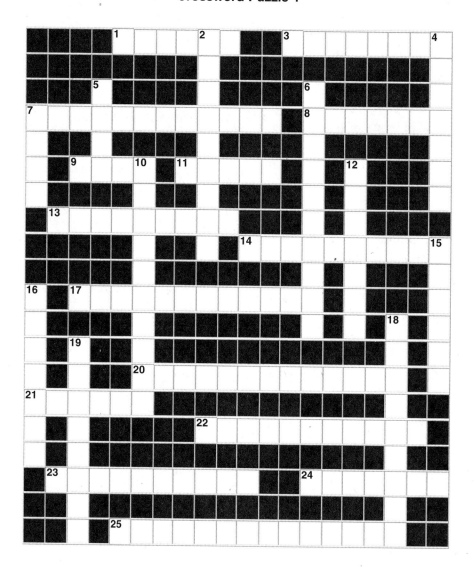

Across

1. Group of organs functioning together
3. Closely apposed sheets of bone tissue in compact bone
7. Organelles associated with manufacture of adenosine triphosphate
8. Largest and most conspicuous organelle in the cell
9. Smallest unit of organization in the body
11. Somewhat independent part that performs a specific function or functions
13. Chief nucleoprotein in the nondividing nucleoplasm
14. White blood cell that increases in numbers during an immune response
17. Three-dimensional system of support within the cell
20. Type of intermediate filament with major role in intercellular junctions
21. Structure formed by cell groups with similar characteristics of shape and function
22. Immature connective tissue formed during initial repair
23. Filamentous daughter chromosomes joined at the centromere during cell division
24. Specialized connective tissue composed of fat, little matrix, and adipocytes
25. Along with calcium, main inorganic crystal in enamel, bone, dentin, and cementum

Down

2. Superficial layers of skin
4. Type of protein fiber in connective tissue composed of microfilaments
5. Rigid connective tissue
6. Metabolically inert substances or transient structures within the cell
7. White blood cell similar to basophil that is also involved in allergic responses
10. Second most common white blood cell in the blood
12. Part of cell division resulting in two daughter cells identical to the parent cell
15. Small space that surrounds chondrocyte or osteocyte
16. Intermediate protein filament that consists of an opaque waterproof substance
18. Intercellular junction found between cells
19. White blood cell that contains granules of histamine and heparin

UNIT III: DENTAL HISTOLOGY

Crossword Puzzle 2

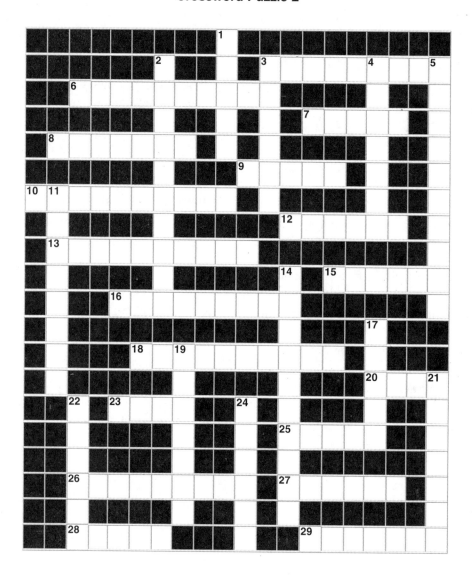

Across

3. Tissue deep to oral mucosa composed of loose connective tissue

6. Joined matrix pieces forming lattice in cancellous bone

7. Tissue fluid that drains from the surrounding region into lymphatic vessels

8. Initially formed bone matrix

9. Central opening where saliva is deposited after production by secretory cells

10. Mature osteoblasts entrapped in bone matrix

12. Respiratory mucosal cells that produce mucus to keep mucosa moist

13. Network of vessels that collect and transport lymph linking the lymph nodes

15. Hard tooth tissue loss from demineralization by cariogenic bacteria

16. Blood cell fragments that function in clotting mechanism

18. Dense connective tissue layer on outer part of bone

20. Extension or "peg" of the epithelium into connective tissue in microscopic section

23. Passageway that allows glandular secretion to be emptied directly into location of use

25. Large inner part of certain glands

26. Dense connective tissue in both dermis and lamina propria

27. Secretion from salivary glands that lubricates and cleanses oral cavity

28. Bundle of neural processes outside the central nervous system

29. Localized macules of pigmentation

Down

1. Depression on one side of the lymph node

2. Grooves associated with lines of Retzius in enamel

3. Connective tissue that divides inner part of certain glands

4. Connective tissue that surrounds outer part of entire gland or lesion

5. Cells that differentiate from preameloblasts forming enamel during amelogenesis

11. Epithelium that stands away from the tooth creating a gingival sulcus

14. Cells that function in resorption of bone

17. Nostril of nose

19. Incremental lines located in histologic preparations of mature enamel

21. Hard tooth tissue loss through chemical means not involving bacteria

22. Functional cellular component of the nervous system

24. Extracellular substance that serves as framework for later calcification

UNIT III: DENTAL HISTOLOGY

Crossword Puzzle 3

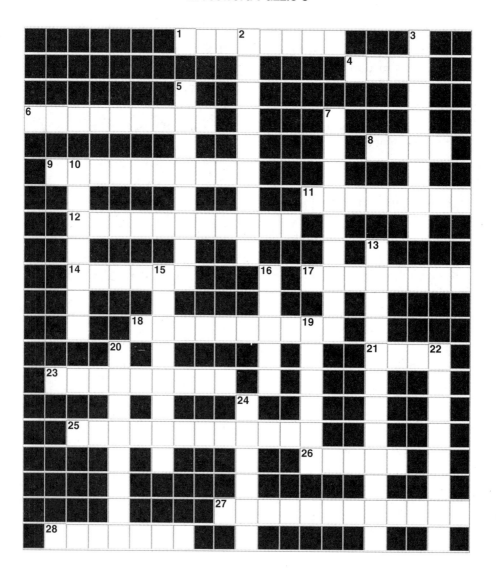

Across

1. Inflammation of pulp

4. Soft innermost connective tissue in both the crown and root

6. Hard tooth tissue loss by mastication or parafunctional habits

8. Crystalline structural units of hardest tissue that gives teeth the bright white look

9. Layered formation of firm or hard tissue such as enamel, dentin, or cementum

11. Surrounds the teeth for support and attaches the teeth to the alveoli

12. Incremental lines or bands of von Ebner in mature dentin

14. Opening or foramen from the pulp at apex

17. Socket of tooth

18. Cancellous bone located between alveolar bone proper and plates of cortical bone

21. Imbrication lines in dentin demonstrating disturbance in body metabolism

23. Extra openings usually located on the lateral parts of the roots

25. Appositional growth of enamel matrix by ameloblasts

26. Microscopic dark brushes in enamel with bases near the dentinoenamel junction

27. Layer of dentin around the outer pulpal wall

28. Part of the tooth that contains the mass of pulp

Down

2. Dentin matrix laid down by appositional growth by the odontoblasts

3. Microscopic enamel feature of short dentinal tubules near the dentinoenamel junction

5. Plates of compact bone on the facial and lingual surfaces of the alveolar process

7. Part of the pulp located in the root area of the tooth

10. Dentin formed in a tooth before the completion of the apical foramen

13. Supporting hard or soft dental tissue for the tooth

15. Hard tooth tissue loss by friction from toothbrushing or toothpaste

16. Found within dentinal tubule in dentin

19. Smooth microscopic lines in cartilage, bone, or cementum caused by appositional growth

20. Outermost layer of root of a tooth

22. Accentuated incremental line of Retzius or contour line of Owen from birth process

24. Hard inner layer of the crown of a tooth overlying pulp

UNIT IV: DENTAL ANATOMY

Crossword Puzzle 1

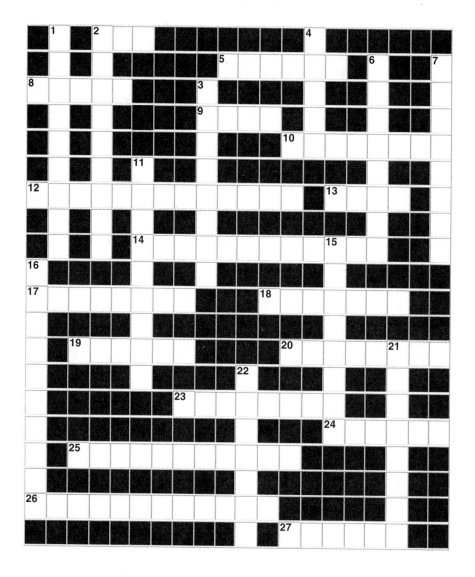

Across

2. Small lateral incisor or third molar crown due to partial microdontia

5. Palmer Notation _____

8. Mythologic nighttime creature that takes shed primary teeth leaving cold hard cash

9. Type of angle formed by lines created at junction of two crown surfaces

10. Rounded enamel extensions on anterior incisal ridge as noted from labial or lingual

12. Tooth designation system using a two-digit code

13. Imaginary line representing a long line of a tooth that bisects the cervical line

14. Crown or root(s) that show angular distortion

17. Rounded raised borders on mesial and distal parts of lingual surface of anteriors

18. Older dental term for canines with much thanks to our tail-wagging friends

19. Surface of a tooth closest to midline

20. Masticatory surface of posteriors

23. Vertically oriented and labially placed bony ridges of the alveolar process in both jaws

24. Surface of tooth farthest away from midline

25. Indentations on surface of the root or roots

26. Secondary groove on lingual surface of anteriors and occlusal table on posteriors

27. Division of a crown surface or root into three parts

Down

1. Division of each dental arch into two parts with four for entire dentition

2. Second dentition noted in oral cavity; also considered *adult teeth*

3. Part of root visible to the clinician

4. Depression on lingual surface of anteriors or occlusal table of posteriors

6. Complete displacement of the tooth from the socket caused by extensive trauma

7. Open contact existing between maxillary central incisors

11. Absence of a single tooth or multiple teeth because of lack of initiation

15. Unerupted or partially erupted tooth positioned against an oral structure

16. Spaces formed from the curvatures where two teeth in the same arch contact

21. Division of each dental arch into three parts based on midline

22. Linear elevation or ridge on masticatory surface of newly erupted incisors

UNIT IV: DENTAL ANATOMY

Crossword Puzzle 2

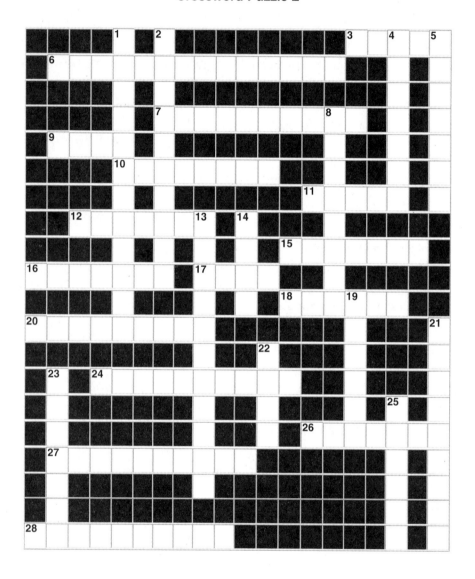

Across

3. Situation in which entire posterior quadrant functions during lateral occlusion

6. Movements of the mandible that are not within the usual patterns

7. Moving lower jaw forward

9. Temporomandibular joint part between temporal bone and mandibular condyle

10. Ridge running mesiodistally in the cervical one-third of the buccal crown surface

11. Natural movement of all of the teeth over time toward the midline of the oral cavity

12. Parafunctional habit of grinding teeth that can sound like a jet taking off

15. First dentition; also known as *deciduous dentition*

16. Side to which the mandible has been moved during lateral occlusion

17. Terminal plane with primary mandibular second molar mesial to the maxillary molar

18. Space when primary molars are shed for making room for permanent premolars

20. Contralateral side of the arch from working side during lateral occlusion

24. Prominent mandible with normal or even retrusive maxilla and concave profile

26. End point of closure of the mandible with it in its most retruded position

27. Lowering of lower jaw

28. Moving lower jaw backward

Down

1. Failure to have overall ideal form of the dentition while in centric occlusion

2. Cusps that function during centric occlusion

4. Maxillary dental arch facially overhangs the mandibular arch

5. Specific spaces between certain primary teeth

8. Situation in which the maxillary incisors overlap the mandibular incisors

13. Facial profile in centric occlusion with slightly protruded jaws

14. Plane where maxillary arch is convex occlusally and mandibular arch concave

19. Concave curve that results when a frontal section is taken through each molar set

21. Parafunctional habit with teeth held in centric occlusion for long periods

22. Situation in which the canine is the only tooth in function during lateral occlusion

23. Bony projection off posterior and superior borders of the mandibular ramus

25. What can occur to the periodontium and that can result from occlusal disharmony

PART 3: UNIT WORD SEARCH PUZZLES

UNIT I: OROFACIAL STRUCTURES

Words to Find

ALA
ANGLE
APEX
ARTICULATING
BUCCAL
COMMISSURE
CONDYLE
CORONOID
FRONTAL
HYOID

INFRAORBITAL
LABIOMENTAL
LARYNX
LYMPH
MANDIBLE
MASSETER
MENTAL
NARIS
NASAL
NOSE

ORBIT
PARATHYROID
PAROTID
PHILTRUM
PROPORTIONS
RAMUS
ROOT
STERNOCLEIDOMASTOID
SUBLINGUAL
SUBMANDIBULAR

SUBMENTAL
SULCUS
SYMPHYSIS
TEMPOROMANDIBULAR
THYROID
TUBERCLE
VERMILION
ZYGOMATIC

Word Search Puzzle 1

```
L A R Y N X S K P R O P O R T I O N S I
S R D O G Z H L A T N O R F T O O R D R
I Y A I R E L C R E B U T S Y L W I A Y
S S E L O D I O R Y H T A R A P O L L D
Y S L A U Y H N O S E H Q L O T U A I E
H I Y T G B H P C U S P A A S B T O R S
P R D N E J I I M U Y I L A I I R U U B
M A N E N W T D B Y B A M D B Y S C L M
Y N O M B A J L N A L O N R H S L A Q A
S H C B M A I E L A D A O T I U B V L S
C J U O N F O L I M A L M S I G A R S
C I G G K S M E B R O M N O X T B V E
T Y L U E A T L U F I O R M B N E X B T
Z E A Z N N C S N L C D E O E U P P J E
L L V F K O U I U A A N N M P A C X A R
M D I O N O R O C M T S B A R M Y C Y R
A M U R T L I H P A A U A O M I E M A L
P I E A X Q M E L I S R T N J A N T U L
E T C Z E R A H A R T I C U L A T I N G
S N O I L I M R E V D T I B R O G P Z V
```

UNIT I: OROFACIAL STRUCTURES

Words to Find

ALVEOLAR
ALVEOLUS
ANTERIOR
CARUNCLE
CECUM
DORSAL
EXOSTOSES
FACIAL
FAUCES
FAUCIAL
FILIFORM
FIMBRIATA

FOLIATE
FORDYCE
FORNIX
FUNGIFORM
GINGIVA
INCISORS
LABIAL
LINGUAL
MASTICATION
MELANIN
MOLARS
MUCOBUCCAL

MUCOGINGIVAL
MUCOSA
NASOPHARYNX
OROPHARYNX
PAROTID
PERIODONTAL
PERMANENT
POSTERIOR
PREMOLARS
PRIMARY
PTERYGOMANDIBULAR
PULP

RAPHE
RETROMOLAR
SUBMANDIBULAR
TASTE
TERMINALIS
TONSIL
TORUS
TUBEROSITY
UVULA
VENTRAL
VESTIBULES

Word Search Puzzle 2

```
T  S  R  O  S  I  C  N  I  F  P  R  I  M  A  R  Y  F  V  T
S  L  D  E  G  N  L  M  I  L  V  S  A  Q  R  R  R  O  E  O
R  H  A  G  L  A  O  M  R  E  A  S  U  O  W  A  A  L  N  N
A  N  O  V  I  C  B  I  S  O  O  U  I  L  L  P  I  T  S
L  Y  U  B  I  R  N  T  T  C  F  R  G  U  O  O  H  A  R  I
O  Y  A  L  I  G  I  U  U  A  E  I  B  N  U  E  E  T  A  L
M  L  T  A  A  B  N  M  R  T  C  I  L  X  I  V  V  E  L  S
E  X  T  I  U  C  L  I  N  A  D  I  W  I  S  L  U  L  I  O
R  A  N  L  S  A  C  A  G  N  C  N  T  U  F  A  J  L  A  L
P  T  E  Y  I  O  D  U  A  O  A  E  B  S  A  T  A  S  A  R
Z  S  N  C  R  O  R  M  B  S  C  M  C  W  A  N  X  T  A  M
F  R  U  E  R  A  O  E  O  O  A  U  E  U  I  M  N  L  R  Y
P  A  O  S  N  G  H  P  B  N  C  X  M  M  M  O  O  O  F  R
F  G  A  I  Y  A  H  P  D  U  O  U  R  U  D  M  F  O  P  M
F  L  I  R  R  A  M  I  O  S  T  E  M  O  O  I  R  A  F  E
W  A  E  N  R  E  B  R  T  R  T  S  I  R  G  D  R  O  A  L
F  T  U  Y  G  U  T  O  E  A  O  R  T  N  Y  O  R  P  C  A
P  A  N  C  L  I  S  S  S  P  E  E  U  C  T  N  U  E  I  N
O  X  T  A  E  E  V  T  O  P  R  F  E  I  I  L  N  F  A  I
T  O  R  U  S  S  E  A  T  P  H  S  D  X  P  I  J  H  L  N
```

UNIT II: DENTAL EMBRYOLOGY

Words to Find

AMNIOCENTESIS
BILAMINAR
BLASTOCYST
CAUDAL
CEPHALIC
CLEAVAGE
CLOACAL
CONGENITAL
DISC

ECTODERM
EMBRYO
ENDODERM
EPIBLAST
FERTILIZATION
FETUS
FOLDING
FUSION
HYPOBLAST

INDUCTION
KARYOTYPE
MATURATION
MEIOSIS
MESODERM
MITOSIS
MORPHOLOGY
NEUROECTODERM
PRENATAL

PRIMORDIUM
SOMITES
SYMMETRY
TERATOGENS
TRILAMINAR
ZYGOTE

Word Search Puzzle 1

```
Q F E V U D C L L S F D C L E A V A G E
A B P T X S F L M E S O D E R M S M L S
Q E I R S Y M M E T R Y B I H N R A I N
C C B I B L A S T O C Y S T E E T S O S
L T L L M I T O S I S G R G D I E I U W
O O A A W R C L V S J S O O N T T T E P
A D S M Y J A N I A E T T E N C E T R H
C E T I W D G S G T A C G E U F F D P Z
A R M N U B O D I R E N C D E P E Q R C
L M E A C I L M E O O O N C H I R J E R
M G C R E U O T R C I I P M Y D T K N O
J A B M F S Y U C N H K R O P S I U A E
F C T I X O E W M U U A I R O A L E T M
U E M U L N L A J H R R M P B B I N A B
S P D R R A Z D O Q I Y O H L X Z D L R
I H J H A A M Y I U Y O R O A S A O U Y
O A D G L Z T I G N U T D L S F T D H O
N L J I R D L I N O G Y I O T F I E Z T
K I U J S S V F O A T P U G C L O R Q B
B C Q T O C K O H N R E M Y L K N M X V
```

UNIT II: DENTAL EMBRYOLOGY

Words to Find

APPOSITION
BELL
BUD
CEMENTOBLASTS
CEMENTOCYTES
CEMENTOID
DILACERATION
ECTODERM

ECTOMESENCHYME
FUSION
GEMINATION
INDUCTION
INITIATION
MACRODONTIA
MALASSEZ
MATRIX

MEMBRANE
MICRODONTIA
MORPHOGENESIS
NONSUCCEDANEOUS
ODONTOBLASTS
ODONTOCLASTS
ORGAN
PEARL

PREAMELOBLASTS
PREDENTIN
REPOLARIZATION
RESORPTION
SHEATH
SUCCEDANEOUS
SUPERNUMERARY

Word Search Puzzle 2

```
W C X O O X X L C E M E N T O C Y T E S
M M A L A S S E Z E N N N N S N S S V X
I B S F U S I O N I O O O I O T U K I E
C R E S Y G K A T I I I S I S O Y R O S
R Z X L P J R N T T T E T A E F T O T O
O F P Q L B E A I A N A L N O A S S B L
D C C L M D N S I E Z B A E M N A X R N
O E Z E E I O T G I O D V C H L W A A S
N M M R M P I O R L E E N T B F E G O U
T E P E P N H A E C Z O A O M P R I D P
I N G A I P L M C G I E T M A O R N O E
A T D D R O A U Q T H N K E C C E D N R
R O U O P E S J A S O O B S R E S U T N
O B M E R N L R H D E H M E O M O C O U
E L R P O Q E S O T Y Q R N D E R T C M
K A W N E C E B M Q N D M C O N P I L E
I S R C A E C T O D E R M H N T T O A R
R T U L N E Q L J M D F B Y T O I N S A
A S I S D P B I O Y P C U M I I O F T R
C D J A S U W R V E E R T E A D N H S Y
```

UNIT III: DENTAL HISTOLOGY

Words to Find

CELL
CENTROMERE
CENTROSOME
CHROMATIDS
CHROMATIN
CHROMOSOMES
CYTOPLASM
CYTOSKELETON
DESMOSOME

ENDOCYTOSIS
EXOCYTOSIS
HEMIDESMOSOME
HISTOLOGY
INCLUSIONS
INTERPHASE
KERATIN
LYSOSOMES
METAPHASE

MICROFILAMENTS
MICROTUBULES
MITOCHONDRIA
MITOSIS
NUCLEOLUS
NUCLEOPLASM
NUCLEUS
ORGAN
PHAGOCYTOSIS

PROPHASE
RIBOSOMES
SYSTEM
TELOPHASE
TISSUE
TONOFILAMENTS
VACUOLES

Word Search Puzzle 1

```
M I M E K W Q Q P H A G O C Y T O S I S
I J E X K U N W E E M S S S S S S E A A
T G T D B E U U S S I E I D S T S E I E
O D A I I K S A A S M S I U N A Q R M S
S M P K K S H L O O O T L E H S D O E M
I M H L I P P T S A O M P E N S L S J
S J A T O O Y O Y M E A O M O O O A E S
M I S L T C M C O L L R O H R U L M T N
I N E Y O O O R C I P S C T C P O N I S
C T C X R D H U F Y O O N A O S E T N V
R E E H N C N O X M T E V E O M A O W E
O R C E P H R G S I C O L M A R I L R C
T P I C F C I E M N U C S L E S L E T H
U H G B I N D S A U U E I K U L M N Z R
B A S M O I U G T N D F I L E O S S T O
U S M S M S R C B O O L C C R L F Y O M
L E R E W O O M L N L N R T H P E S A A
E V H O O Q Z M O E I O N M B N H T D T
S D D Z D I Q T E C U E G R T H J E O I
L Y S O S O M E S S C S X Y Z N V M O N
```

UNIT III: DENTAL HISTOLOGY

Words to Find

ADIPOSE
APPOSITIONAL
BASOPHIL
BONE
CANALICULI
CARTILAGE
CHONDROBLASTS
CHONDROCYTES

COLLAGEN
DERMIS
ELASTIC
ENDOSTEUM
ENDOTHELIUM
EOSINOPHIL
EPIDERMIS
EPITHELIUM

FIBROBLAST
GRANULATION
HAVERSIAN
HEMIDESMOSOMES
HYDROXYAPATITE
IMMUNOGEN
IMMUNOGLOBULIN
INTERSTITIAL

KERATIN
LACUNA
LAMELLAE
LYMPHOCYTE
MACROPHAGE
MAST

Word Search Puzzle 2

```
N E S J X J V B O N E C A R T I L A G E
M A S T E P I T H E L I U M L A C U N A
U J E I J C B D L M X B D R O Z T Z I C
W I L M J H E I U L A M E L L A E L F W
I J A M O O I M M U N O G L O B U L I N
H Z S U E N Q K V M M E P I D E R M I S
I C T N A D D E R M I S D R O K X Y G H
T L I O P R C B F O F I B R O B L A S T
G D C G P O I I F A M A C R O P H A G E
G B G E O C H E M I D E S M O S O M E S
E B R N S Y Q I W E N D O T H E L I U M
O U A H I T W C H O N D R O B L A S T S
S B N A T E Q C P V A J C O L L A G E N
I A U V I S J A D I P O S E Z S V P U C
N S L E O Y G J D S D D R K E R A T I N
O O A R N Q E W U F L Y M P H O C Y T E
P P T S A W Z S I N T E R S T I T I A L
H H I I L K C U O B I E N D O S T E U M
I I O A R F H Y D R O X Y A P A T I T E
L L N N W J Q B B I C A N A L I C U L I
```

UNIT III: DENTAL HISTOLOGY

Words to Find

ENDOCHONDRAL
INTRAMEMBRANOUS
MATRIX
MONOCYTE
NERVE
NEURON
NEUTROPHIL

ODONTOCLAST
OSSIFICATION
OSTEOBLASTS
OSTEOCLAST
OSTEOCYTES
OSTEOID
OSTEONS

PAPILLARY
PERICHONDRIUM
PERIOSTEUM
PLASMA
PLATELETS
RETE
RETICULAR

SQUAMES
SUBMUCOSA
SYNAPSE
TONOFILAMENTS
TRABECULAE

Word Search Puzzle 3

```
U S P L A S M A E L L I C O I O H X L Z
B U T F Z M F W P Y R X F Z A T C D N L
J B O Y Y W N D L H W F J R S T I O A X
I M N R V S Y N A P S E F A H O I R S M
V U O E F K F O T J I W L O E T D K U B
P C F T L I B X E S H C T T A N U E A K
L O I I Z N S O L D O W S C O A T W B U
T S L C G T P F E E I O I H W S V T P Z
L A A U V R G W T E P F C H O O S F E G
B C M L O A S S S C I O S I E A E P R X
L T E A S M O P V S D C R T L V O A I N
E R N R T E N L S N K E Y C R N S P C E
W A T G E M B O E R P C O E O Z T I H U
O B S S O B D R I D O T N Z O F E L O T
N E X Q B R R G X N N C W M S B O L N R
E C K U L A P P O O M V K A T V C A D O
U U B A A N K M D A V E C T E K Y R R P
R L R M S O M O D J T P E R O G T Y I H
O A J E T U N K W E A J S I N K E W U I
N E T S S S F K R I C U H X S B S X M L
```

UNIT III: DENTAL HISTOLOGY

Words to Find

AFFERENT
CAPSULE
COLLOID
DENTOGINGIVAL
DUCT
EFFERENT
ENDOCRINE
EXOCRINE
FIBROBLAST
FOLLICLES

GERMINAL
GINGIVITIS
GOBLET
GOITER
GRANULATION
HILUS
HYPERKERATINIZED
JUNCTIONAL
KERATIN
KERATOHYALINE

LOBES
LOBULES
LUMEN
LYMPH
MASTICATORY
MELANIN
MUCOGINGIVAL
MUCOPERIOSTEUM
MUCOSA
NODES

PERIODONTITIS
PRICKLE
RECESSION
STIPPLING
SULCULAR
SULCUS
TASTE

Word Search Puzzle 4

```
N O D E S E G V K Y Q K A O S U L C U S
A P C K O N P E H K A U R F E L E I T P
H R O H D D M Z R G E E S N F N Y S Y T
A I L H K O U U D M T R I L I E A M C D
E C L Z L C H D C I I R A L O L R U P G
T K O U I R Y E O O C N A T B B D E N H
A L I T S I P G G O P Y A O I S E I N N
P E D D T N E Y X O H E R L E N L S O T
E S W E A E R E E O B B R L M P B I Z L
R E M N S M K Z T A I L C I P G S S A N
I G A T T U E A M F T I E I O S T V O S
O I S O E D R L P S L E T T E S I I E Z
D N T G I E A V A L U S Z C N G T L W A
O G I I K C T V O N I L E L N A U E S V
N I C N E A I F X G I R C I L B Z O U V
T V A G X P N I A J A N G U O A C L Y M
I I T I V S I M O M J O N L L U P U U N
T T O V F U Z S H N C A M W M A I M Z L
I I R A D L E P B U R M E F F E R E N T
S S Y L X E D Z M G J U N C T I O N A L
```

UNIT III: DENTAL HISTOLOGY

Words to Find

ABFRACTION
ABRASION
AMELOBLAST
AMELOGENESIS
ATTRITION
CARIES
DEMILUNE

EROSION
LYMPHADENOPATHY
LYMPHATICS
MUCOCELE
MUCOSEROUS
MYOEPITHELIAL
NARIS

PARATHYROID
PERIKYMATA
RANULA
RETZIUS
SALIVA
SECRETORY
SEPTUM

SINUSITIS
THYROGLOSSAL
THYROID
THYROXINE
TONSILS
TRABECULAE
XEROSTOMIA

Word Search Puzzle 5

```
I  B  W  S  T  H  Y  R  O  X  I  N  E  T  T  P  E  Z  P  B
S  A  B  F  R  A  C  T  I  O  N  N  K  F  S  K  Z  E  S  S
L  C  A  R  I  E  S  I  L  H  O  G  X  Z  V  I  A  U  I  A
P  A  R  A  T  H  Y  R  O  I  D  Y  E  U  Y  L  O  S  T  T
F  G  Y  L  S  I  N  U  S  I  T  I  S  H  U  R  E  A  S  N
G  D  Y  W  H  G  I  A  M  P  S  K  T  C  E  N  M  A  O  W
Y  E  D  M  U  U  R  X  L  R  N  A  E  S  E  Y  L  I  A  S
M  M  S  U  B  U  M  E  Y  P  B  O  G  K  B  T  D  C  D
U  I  A  E  A  J  C  Y  R  O  A  C  O  I  O  I  S  I  I  S
C  L  L  P  N  Z  W  O  N  R  U  L  R  L  R  V  T  O  U  N
O  U  I  T  I  W  T  E  T  M  E  E  E  T  D  A  R  I  O  C
C  N  V  U  U  E  D  P  E  M  P  M  T  F  H  Y  Z  I  D  L
E  E  A  M  R  A  Q  I  A  U  A  A  R  P  H  T  S  K  Q  F
L  H  T  C  H  U  R  T  Z  U  B  P  M  T  E  O  W  M  M  X
E  G  E  P  Y  G  A  H  R  F  R  Y  U  R  R  U  Q  I  G  W
P  S  M  F  Z  X  N  E  O  Y  L  W  G  E  R  G  D  A  N  T
X  Y  U  B  Z  A  U  L  E  F  X  E  R  O  S  T  O  M  I  A
L  K  N  K  S  F  L  I  C  Q  L  L  E  T  O  N  S  I  L  S
I  E  U  V  W  F  A  A  T  H  Y  R  O  G  L  O  S  S  A  L
P  H  T  B  F  V  N  L  N  A  R  I  S  B  F  W  H  S  U  Q
```

UNIT III: DENTAL HISTOLOGY

Words to Find

ACCESSORY
ALVEOLUS
APICAL
APPOSITION
ARREST
ATTRITION
CANALICULI
CEMENTICLES
CEMENTOBLASTS
CEMENTOCYTES
CEMENTOGENESIS

CEMENTOID
CEMENTUM
CHAMBER
CIRCUMPULPAL
DENTIN
DENTINOGENESIS
EDENTULOUS
FLUID
GLOBULAR
HYPERCEMENTOSIS
HYPERSENSITIVITY

IMBRICATION
INTERGLOBULAR
INTERTUBULAR
MANTLE
NEONATAL
ODONTOBLASTS
OWEN
PERIODONTIUM
PERITUBULAR
PREDENTIN
PRIMARY

PRINCIPAL
PULP
PULPITIS
RADICULAR
SECONDARY
STONES
TERTIARY
TRABECULAR
TUBULES

Word Search Puzzle 6

```
A T T A T Q M P N T G K O I B S A D C C
R E U L C P A U E R D A W M P T T B E H
R R B V E R N L O A E P E B R O T U M A
E T U E M I T P N B N I N R I N R B E M
S I L O E N L I A E T C H I M E I H N B
T A E L N C E T T C I A Y C A S T Z T E
C R S U T I C I A U N L P A R H I C U R
E Y P S O P E S L L O I E T Y Y O E M C
M P E C I A M E I A G N R I O P N M P E
E E R I D L E V N R E T S O D E K E R M
N R I R K C N E T Z N E E N O C A N E E
T I O C S A T D E R E R N A N E P T D N
I T D U E N O E R A S G S C T M P O E T
C U O M C A G N T D I L I C O E O C N O
L B N P O L E T U I S O T E B N S Y T B
E U T U N I N U B C F B I S L T I T I L
S L I L D C E L U U L U V S A O T E N A
U A U P A U S O L L U L I O S S I S W S
I R M A R L I U A A I A T R T I O Q R T
Y Q X L Y I S S R R D R Y Y S S N E Q S
```

UNIT IV: DENTAL ANATOMY

Words to Find

ANATOMIC	CUSP	INTERPROXIMAL	PERMANENT
AXIS	DECIDUOUS	MASTICATORY	PRIMARY
CEMENTOENAMEL	DENTITION	MESIAL	PROXIMAL
CLINICAL	DISTAL	MIDLINE	QUADRANTS
CONCAVITIES	EMBRASURES	OCCLUSAL	SEXTANTS
CONTACT	INCISAL	OCCLUSION	THIRDS
CONTOUR	INTERNATIONAL	PALMER	UNIVERSAL

Word Search Puzzle 1

```
A I A J G I N T E R P R O X I M A L O Q
T H I R D S T L T L R V F L Y R V S B L
P K L N B C F N T M X U A L U C T H E L
N S O Z A A E G Y D A I O O T N A M B L
I F S T K N V W M C S S T C A C A X A J
C S N Z A A U E O E O N T T C N K N I L
T O V M B T N T M K O N X I E L O X A S
C C R P S O I G E C V E C O C I U M L C
H E U Q K M V S J N S O T A T A I S Y E
P N W S K I E D J Q D N C A V X T Q A L
L R L R P C R B U E E I N C O I N O A L
W V I E R A S Q K M M R S R L B T C R S
Z C N M D L A U E R E B P T C U I I U Y
B J C V A H L C C T M P R V A N S O E R
K M I F X R F K N P F C Y A I L U I E S
Q A S F U V Y I A I Z S V L S D U M O I
Z W A U X O N R J M S J C Q I U L E E N
O M L Q U A D R A N T S Z C F A R K D T
X W D E N T I T I O N D E K P Q Z E D D
O H M I D L I N E J H D T W N U Q X S P
```

UNIT IV: DENTAL ANATOMY

Words to Find

ANODONTIA
AVULSION
BICUSPID
BIFURCATED
CARABELLI
CENTRAL
CINGULUM

CUSPIDS
DENTIGEROUS
DIASTEMA
DILACERATION
EMINENCE
FLUTTING
FOSSA

FURCATION
IMPACTED
MAMELONS
MARGINAL
MESIODENS
MULBERRY
MULTIROOTED

PEG
SUPERNUMERARY
SUPPLEMENTAL
TRANSVERSE
TRIANGULAR
TRIFURCATED
TUBERCLES

Word Search Puzzle 2

```
P K A C B B I F U R C A T E D E U F F M
U O A I B T O S T Y E N L W D T D X R D
S I Z N N B I J U S W A U E D I O A E A
F M C G K A D M R P T S D P Y L T A Q
L P J U T G K E A N E O N S Q U A S Y H
U A K L L Z V I E I O R U P G C S G E F
T C W U Y S T M G R S C N N R O R M F V
T T S M N N E L I L I K A U F O V F X E
I E U A O L H T L B H I F D M F X A R I
N D R D P W L Q D U R I Z I Z E X I Y Q
G T O P D U Y A E T R D X L Z I R G Q N
R N U R M F B T N T P C M A M S H A P P
A S M M E U K U T D E A A C P E A I R S
V C U A S R N B I I G R R E N M V C F Y
A U L M I C D E G A S A G R G I U E J L
P S B E O A H R E S L B I A O N L N X C
P P E L D T L C R T Z E N T D E S T D C
X I R O E I C L O E X L A I P N I R D O
I D R N N O B E U M K L L O S C O A D Y
U S Y S S N O S S A B I P N T E N L V X
```

UNIT IV: DENTAL ANATOMY

Words to Find

ABFRACTION
ARTICULAR
BALANCING
BRUXISM
CAPSULE
CENTRIC
CERVICAL
CLENCHING
CONDYLE
CROSSBITE
DEPRESSION

DEVIATION
DISC
DRIFT
ELEVATION
GROUP
INTEROCCLUSAL
LEEWAY
MALOCCLUSION
MESOGNATHIC
OCCLUSION
OVERBITE

OVERJET
PARAFUNCTIONAL
PREMATURE
PRIMARY
PRIMATE
PROGNATHIC
PROTRUSION
RETRACTION
RETROGNATHIC
RISE
SPEE

STEP
SUBLUXATION
SUPPORTING
SYNOVIAL
TEMPOROMANDIBULAR
TERMINAL
TRAUMA
WILSON
WORKING

Word Search Puzzle 3

```
A U F P R I M A T E R E T R A C T I O N
R I N T E R O C C L U S A L W I L S O N
T O N T E M P O R O M A N D I B U L A R
I P G X E L E V A T I O N P R I M A R Y
C O N D Y L E M A L O C C L U S I O N J
U S P M D S U B L U X A T I O N R I S E
L P W O R K I N G B P R O G N A T H I C
A W R X M E S O G N A T H I C D R I F T
R R A E V V C E I U P M T E R M I N A L
H C E O M L E E W A Y D E V I A T I O N
D L P T M A P A R A F U N C T I O N A L
E E B R R X T T O V E R B I T E S T E P
P N A S O O Z U C R O S S B I T E O T J
R C L B C T G Q R T F O C C L U S I O N
E H A R T E R N C E R V I C A L S P E E
S I N U R G N U A V A B F R A C T I O N
S N C X A R D T S T S U P P O R T I N G
I G I I U O I X R I H H S Y N O V I A L
O H N S M U S D Y I O I X O V E R J E T
N W G M A P C Q L I C N C C A P S U L E
```

Introduction

Tooth-drawing assignments emphasize fundamental principles in tooth design, which later have direct practical application in clinical coursework of a student dental professional. It is understood that these initial drawings are most likely to be the student's first attempts at capturing any tooth likeness; therefore the overriding goal is only to encourage accuracy and discernment of the important features of the teeth and hopefully facilitate the recognition of these tooth details. *Thus any overwhelming artistic inclinations are not what is being exercised with these basic technical drawings of the teeth.*

It is important to also note that these drawings are only two-dimensional and are somewhat limited to fundamental outlines and proportions; real specimens in patients' mouths vary considerably. However, these drawings will serve to help create mental pictures of teeth in their ideal and composite state using each standard view of the individual tooth. Later, these mental images can be called upon during clinical situations.

Directions

Step 1. Locate the two blank gridded worksheets in the workbook. Any additional gridded worksheets can be easily scanned and printed for the correct spacing of the grid needed. Correctly label the worksheet at the bottom of the page with the tooth that will be drawn as shown in the smaller professionally drawn figures.

Step 2. Using the attached table of tooth measurements (also included in the associated textbook's Appendix C on tooth measurements), mark off the overall peripheral tooth measurements for each of the gridded view boxes of the tooth. Note that the grid of the blank worksheet is larger than that shown with the professionally drawn tooth outlines to better enable the student to have room to work. Each square of grid equates to 1 mm of actual dimension, so count off as many squares for each peripheral measurement (such as the mesiodistal diameter) as indicated from the table onto the proper area of the gridded worksheet.

Step 3. To establish crown and root proportions, divide each gridded view box into two parts corresponding to these two measurements, except for the incisal or occlusal view.

Step 4. To indicate the height of contour, locate the approximate area of contact between the adjacent teeth and the area of greatest convexity on the labial or buccal, lingual, mesial, and distal surfaces (as mentioned in the associated textbook's Unit 3 on dental anatomy).

Step 5. To locate the root axis line (RAL), draw a line that exactly bisects the overall gridded box showing the overall crown and root measurements. The cementoenamel junction (CEJ) will then be bisected by the RAL. The root apex may or may not be located on this RAL, depending on the tooth's apex traits.

Step 6. To locate the center of the cingulum, the midpoint of the incisal ridge, the center of the occlusal table, root apex, or other important feature, divide the crown and root (if included in that particular view box) into imaginary thirds. Then place the cingulum, incisal ridge, occlusal table, or root apex into proper perspective with respect to the other peripheral overall tooth measurements such as the mesiodistal diameter.

Step 7. To complete the crown outline, connect the heights of contour to the incisal ridge or occlusal table, to the CEJ, and to the other heights of contour. Any additional anatomic features such as marginal ridges, depressions, and so forth can be indicated upon completion of the crown outline.

Step 8. To complete the root outline, follow the directions for developing the crown outline with the understanding that the cervical one-third to one-half of the root width generally approximates the cervical width of the crown before it starts to narrow considerably to form the root apex.

Step 9. Shading or stippling of the features may now be added, if desired.

Step 10. A drawing evaluation checklist is also included and can be used by both the student and instructor. Multiple copies of the form may be scanned and printed if needed.

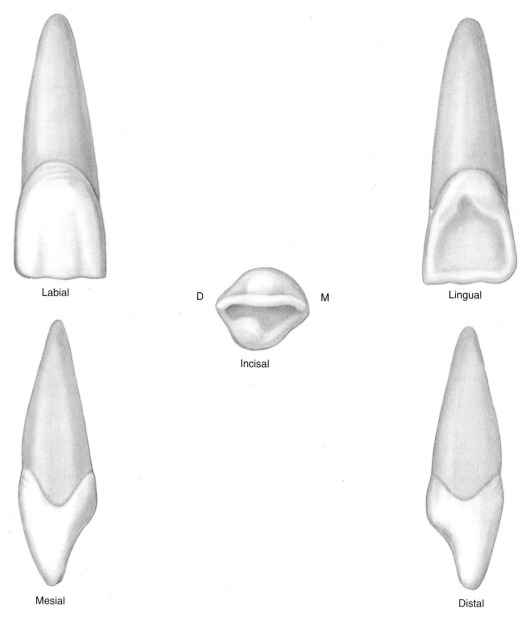

Labial

Lingual

D   M

Incisal

Mesial

Distal

Views of Permanent Maxillary Right Central Incisor

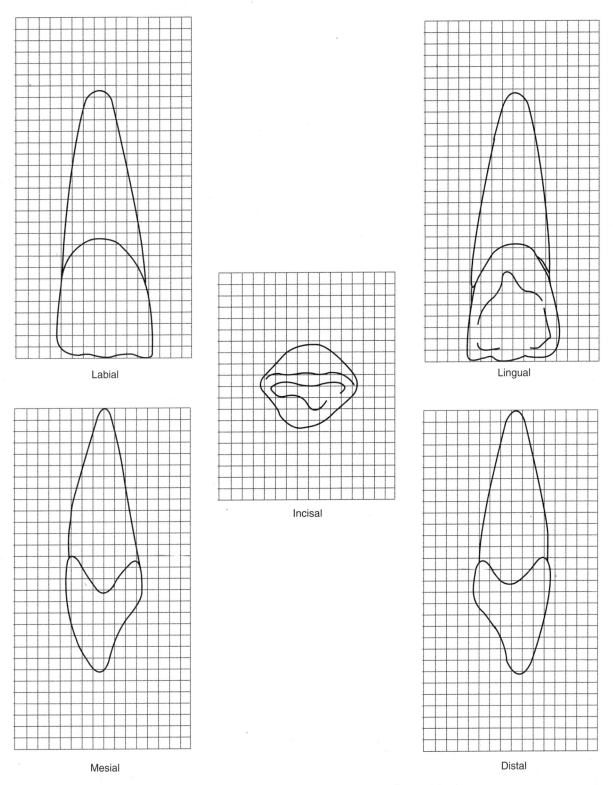

Labial

Incisal

Lingual

Mesial

Distal

Outline Views of Permanent Maxillary Right Central Incisor

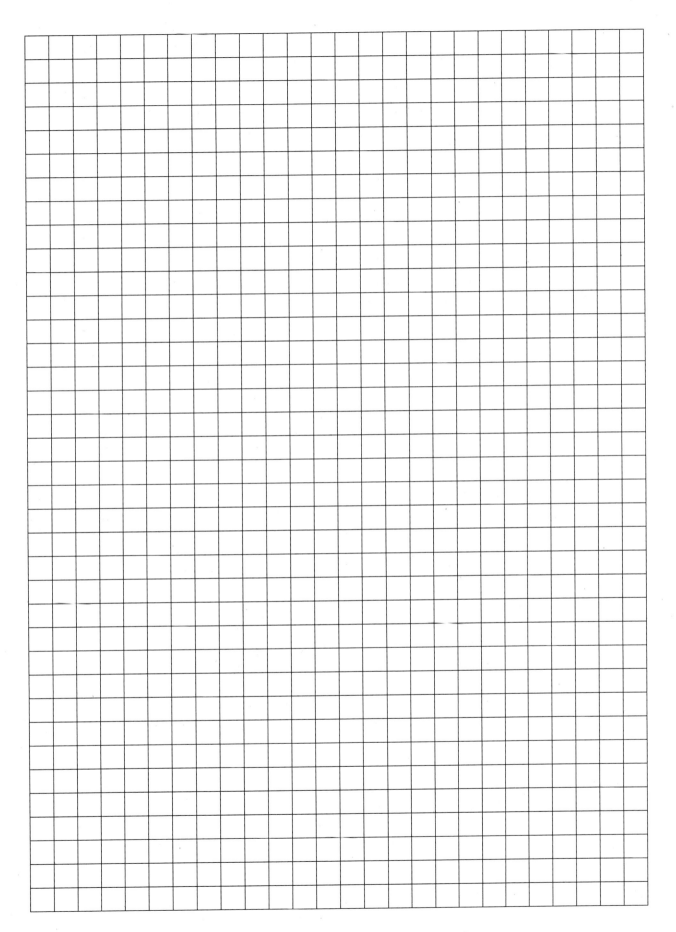

MEASUREMENTS FOR PERMANENT MAXILLARY CENTRAL INCISOR*

Cervico-Incisal Length of Crown	10.5
Length of Root	13.0
Mesiodistal Diameter of Crown	8.5
Mesiodistal Diameter of CEJ	7.0
Labiolingual Diameter	7.0
Labiolingual Diameter of CEJ	6.0
Curvature of CEJ at Mesial	3.5
Curvature of CEJ at Distal	2.5

*In millimeters; adapted from Nelson SJ: *Wheeler's Dental Anatomy, Physiology, and Occlusion.* 10th ed. Philadelphia: Elsevier; 2015.

CHECKLIST FOR PERMANENT MAXILLARY CENTRAL INCISOR

Features Noted	Features Present
Crown Features	
Incisal ridge, incisal angles, cingulum, marginal ridges, lingual fossa	
Pronounced distal offset cingulum and marginal ridges with wide and deep lingual fossa	
Sharper mesioincisal angle and rounder distoincisal angle with more pronounced mesial CEJ curvature	
Height of contour in cervical third	
Mesial contact at incisal third	
Distal contact at junction of incisal and middle thirds	
Root Features	
Single root	
Overall conical shape with no proximal root concavities and rounded apex	

Name _____   Tooth Number/Name _____

Date _____   Instructor Rating _____

DRAWING EVALUATION CHECKLIST

RATING SCALE

Completely Correct = 2 points   Major Error = 0 points
Minor Error = 1 point   Note = NA (nonappropriate)

SELF-EVALUATION RATING

Five Views	Clearly Drawn	Accurate Sizing	General Features Included	Specific Features Included
1. Facial View				
2. Lingual View				
3. Mesial View				
4. Distal View				
5. Incisal/ Occlusal View				

$$\text{Self-Evaluation Rating} = \frac{\text{Points received}}{\text{Points possible}} = \underline{\hspace{2cm}} = \underline{\hspace{2cm}} \%$$

INSTRUCTOR EVALUATION RATING

Five Views	Clearly Drawn	Accurate Sizing	General Features Included	Specific Features Included
1. Facial View				
2. Lingual View				
3. Mesial View				
4. Distal View				
5. Incisal/ Occlusal View				

$$\text{Instructor Evaluation Rating} = \frac{\text{Points received}}{\text{Points possible}} = \underline{\hspace{2cm}} = \underline{\hspace{2cm}} \%$$

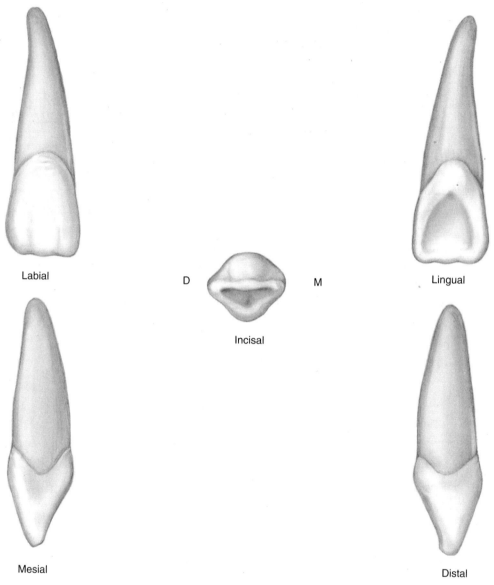

Labial

Lingual

D   M

Incisal

Mesial

Distal

Views of Permanent Maxillary Right Lateral Incisor

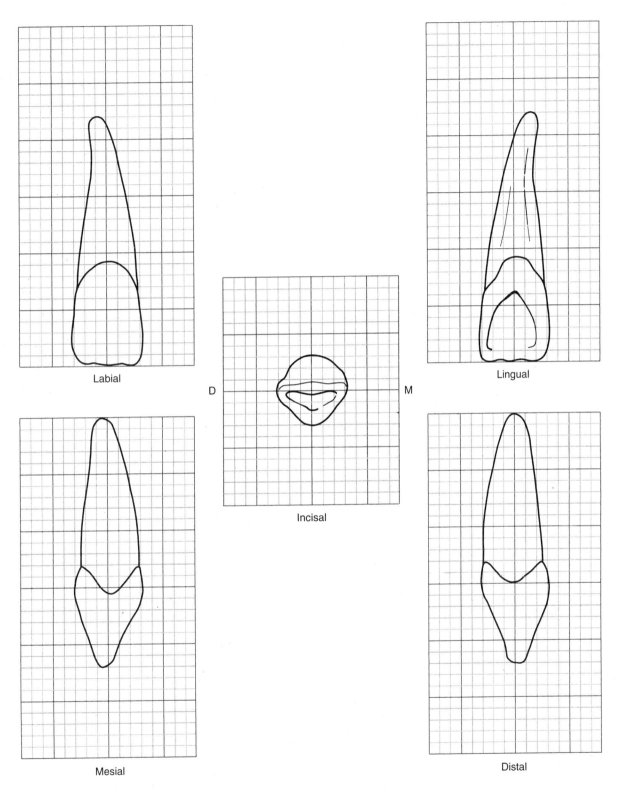

Labial

Lingual

D   M

Incisal

Mesial

Distal

Outline Views of a Permanent Maxillary Right Lateral Incisor

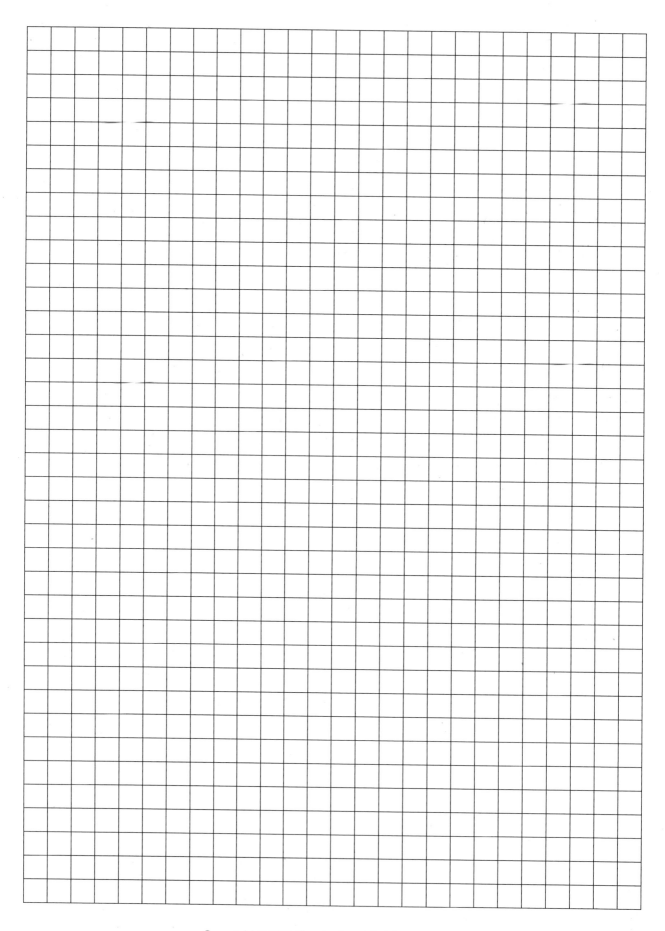

MEASUREMENTS FOR PERMANENT MAXILLARY LATERAL INCISOR*

Cervico-Incisal Length of Crown	9.0
Length of Root	13.0
Mesiodistal Diameter of Crown	6.5
Mesiodistal Diameter of CEJ	5.0
Labiolingual Diameter	6.0
Labiolingual Diameter of CEJ	5.0
Curvature of CEJ at Mesial	3.0
Curvature of CEJ at Distal	2.0

*In millimeters; adapted from Nelson SJ: *Wheeler's Dental Anatomy, Physiology, and Occlusion*. 10th ed. Philadelphia: Elsevier; 2015.

CHECKLIST FOR PERMANENT MAXILLARY LATERAL INCISOR

Features Noted	Features Present
Crown Features	
Incisal ridge, incisal angles, cingulum, marginal ridges, lingual fossa	
Pronounced lingual surface with centered cingulum and prominent marginal ridges	
Sharper mesioincisal angle and rounder distoincisal angle with more pronounced mesial CEJ curvature	
Height of contour in cervical third	
Mesial contact at incisal third	
Distal contact at middle third	
Root Features	
Single root	
Overall conical shape with no proximal root concavities and root curves distally and sharp apex	

Name _____   Tooth Number/Name _____

Date _____   Instructor Rating _____

DRAWING EVALUATION CHECKLIST

RATING SCALE
Completely Correct = 2 points   Major Error = 0 points
Minor Error = 1 point   Note = NA (nonappropriate)

SELF-EVALUATION RATING

Five Views	Clearly Drawn	Accurate Sizing	General Features Included	Specific Features Included
1. Facial View				
2. Lingual View				
3. Mesial View				
4. Distal View				
5. Incisal/ Occlusal View				

Self-Evaluation Rating $= \dfrac{\text{Points received}}{\text{Points possible}} = \rule{2cm}{0.4pt} = \rule{2cm}{0.4pt}$ %

INSTRUCTOR EVALUATION RATING

Five Views	Clearly Drawn	Accurate Sizing	General Features Included	Specific Features Included
1. Facial View				
2. Lingual View				
3. Mesial View				
4. Distal View				
5. Incisal/ Occlusal View				

Instructor Evaluation Rating $= \dfrac{\text{Points received}}{\text{Points possible}} = \rule{2cm}{0.4pt} = \rule{2cm}{0.4pt}$ %

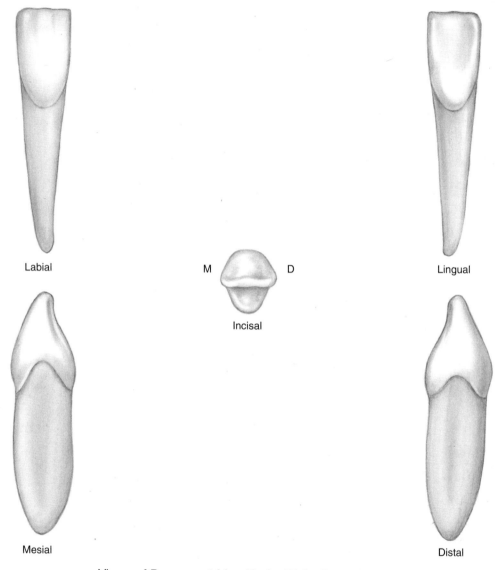

Labial

M   D

Incisal

Lingual

Mesial

Distal

Views of Permanent Mandibular Right Central Incisor

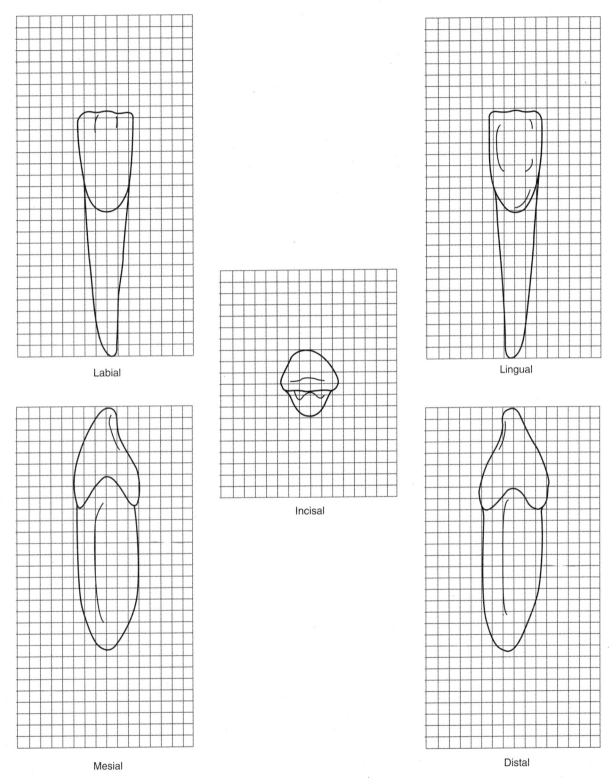

Labial

Lingual

Incisal

Mesial

Distal

Outline Views of Permanent Mandibular Right Central Incisor

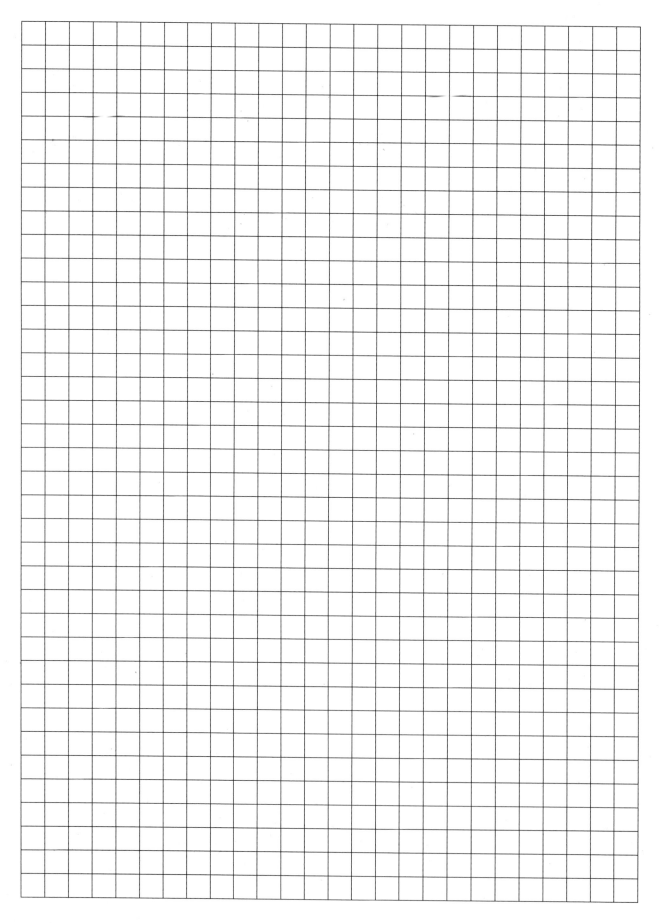

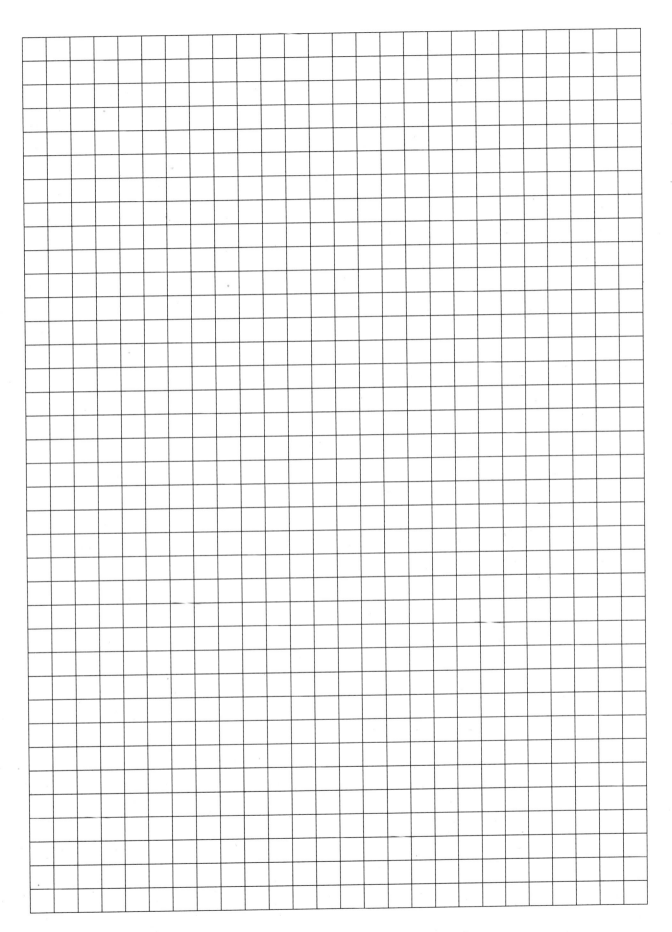

MEASUREMENTS FOR PERMANENT MANDIBULAR CENTRAL INCISOR*

Cervico-Incisal Length of Crown	9.0
Length of Root	12.5
Mesiodistal Diameter of Crown	5.0
Mesiodistal Diameter of CEJ	3.5
Labiolingual Diameter	6.0
Labiolingual Diameter of CEJ	5.3
Curvature of CEJ at Mesial	3.0
Curvature of CEJ at Distal	2.0

*In millimeters; adapted from Nelson SJ: *Wheeler's Dental Anatomy, Physiology, and Occlusion*. 10th ed. Philadelphia: Elsevier; 2015.

CHECKLIST FOR PERMANENT MANDIBULAR CENTRAL INCISOR

Features Noted	Features Present
Crown Features	
Incisal ridge, incisal angles, cingulum, marginal ridges, lingual fossa	
Symmetric with small centered cingulum and less pronounced marginal ridges and lingual fossa	
Sharper mesioincisal angle and rounder distoincisal angle with more pronounced mesial CEJ curvature	
Height of contour in cervical third	
Mesial contact at incisal third	
Distal contact at incisal third	
Root Features	
Single root	
Root longer than crown and pronounced proximal root concavities	

Name _____   Tooth Number/Name _____

Date _____   Instructor Rating _____

DRAWING EVALUATION CHECKLIST

RATING SCALE

Completely Correct = 2 points   Major Error = 0 points
Minor Error = 1 point   Note = NA (nonappropriate)

SELF-EVALUATION RATING

Five Views	Clearly Drawn	Accurate Sizing	General Features Included	Specific Features Included
1. Facial View				
2. Lingual View				
3. Mesial View				
4. Distal View				
5. Incisal/ Occlusal View				

Self-Evaluation Rating = $\frac{\text{Points received}}{\text{Points possible}}$ = _____ = _____ %

INSTRUCTOR EVALUATION RATING

Five Views	Clearly Drawn	Accurate Sizing	General Features Included	Specific Features Included
1. Facial View				
2. Lingual View				
3. Mesial View				
4. Distal View				
5. Incisal/ Occlusal View				

Instructor Evaluation Rating = $\frac{\text{Points received}}{\text{Points possible}}$ = _____ = _____ %

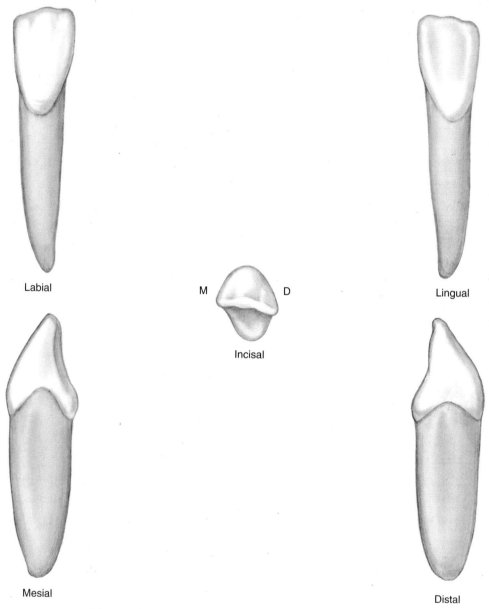

Labial

Lingual

M   D

Incisal

Mesial

Distal

Views of Permanent Mandibular Right Lateral Incisor

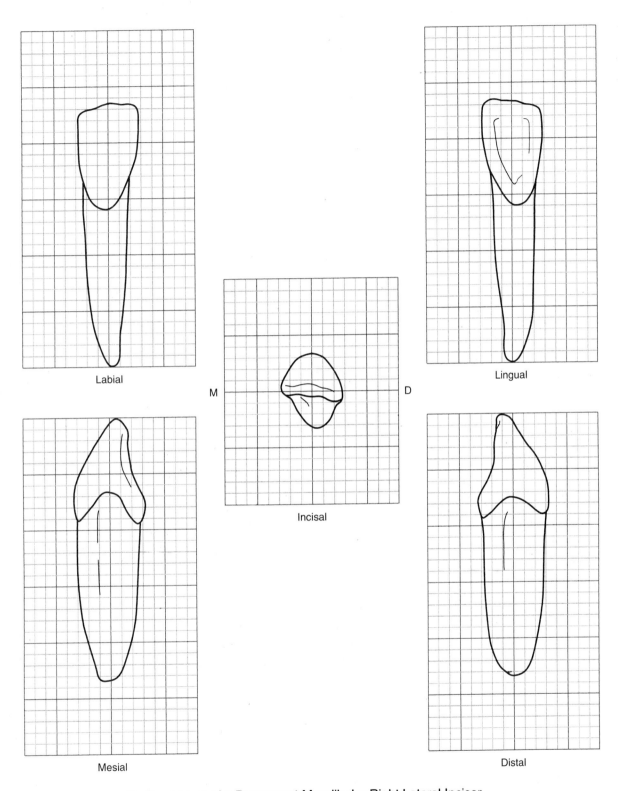

Labial

Lingual

M

D

Incisal

Mesial

Distal

Outline Views of a Permanent Mandibular Right Lateral Incisor

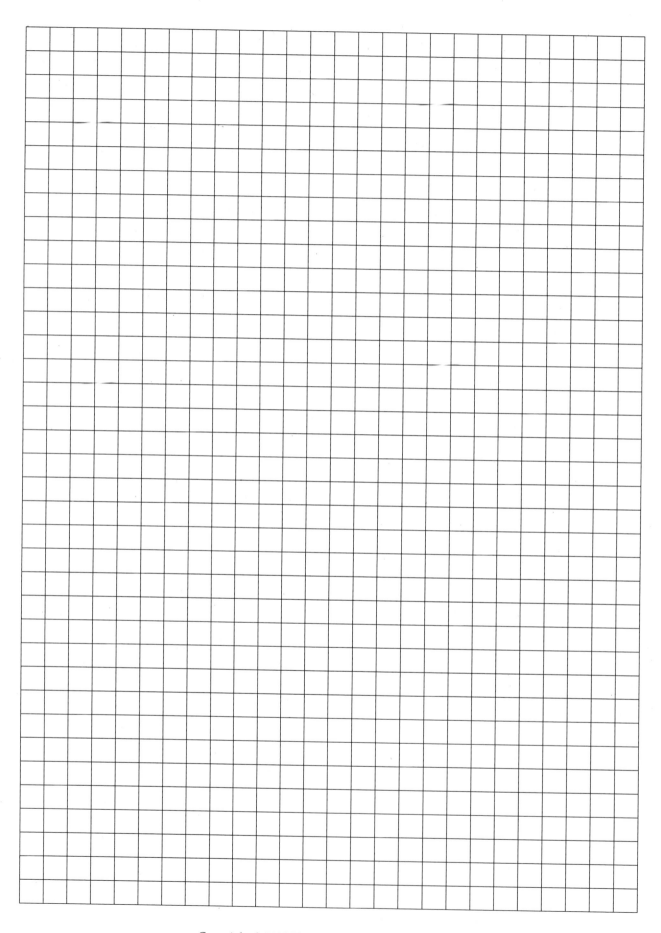

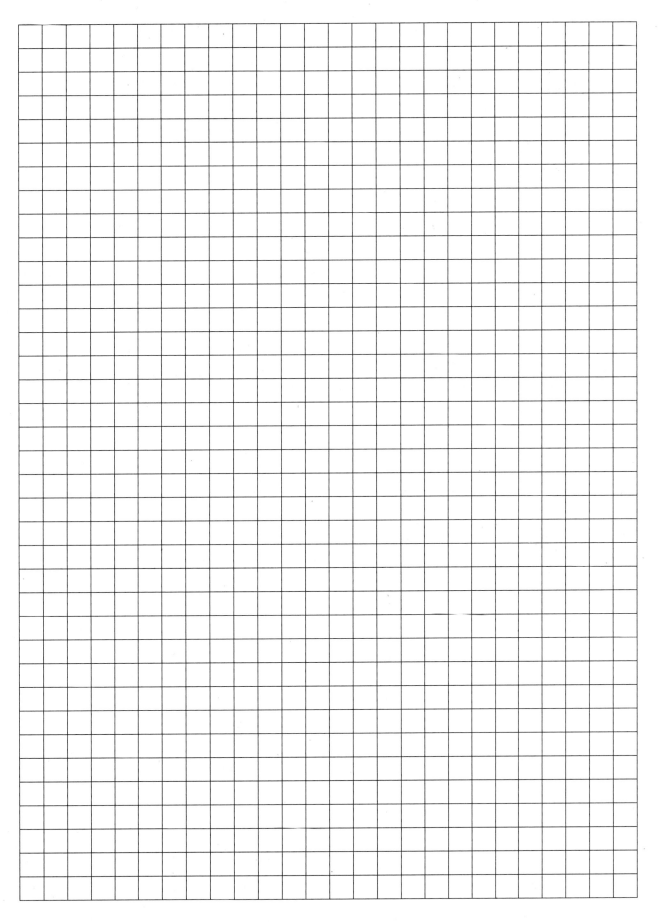

MEASUREMENTS FOR PERMANENT MANDIBULAR LATERAL INCISOR*	
Cervico-Incisal Length of Crown	9.5
Length of Root	14.0
Mesiodistal Diameter of Crown	5.5
Mesiodistal Diameter of CEJ	4.0
Labiolingual Diameter	6.5
Labiolingual Diameter of CEJ	5.8
Curvature of CEJ at Mesial	3.0
Curvature of CEJ at Distal	2.0

*In millimeters; adapted from Nelson SJ: *Wheeler's Dental Anatomy, Physiology, and Occlusion.* 10th ed. Philadelphia: Elsevier; 2015.

CHECKLIST FOR PERMANENT MANDIBULAR LATERAL INCISOR	
Features Noted	**Features Present**
Crown Features	
Incisal ridge, incisal angles, cingulum, marginal ridges, lingual fossa	
Not symmetric and appears twisted distally	
Small distally placed cingulum with mesial marginal ridge longer than distal marginal ridge	
Sharper mesioincisal angle and rounder distoincisal angle with more pronounced mesial CEJ curvature	
Height of contour in cervical third	
Mesial contact at incisal third	
Distal contact at incisal third	
Root Features	
Single root	
Root longer than crown and proximal root concavities	

Name _____   Tooth Number/Name _____

Date _____   Instructor Rating _____

DRAWING EVALUATION CHECKLIST

RATING SCALE
Completely Correct = 2 points   Major Error = 0 points
Minor Error = 1 point   Note = NA (nonappropriate)

SELF-EVALUATION RATING

Five Views	Clearly Drawn	Accurate Sizing	General Features Included	Specific Features Included
1. Facial View				
2. Lingual View				
3. Mesial View				
4. Distal View				
5. Incisal/ Occlusal View				

Self-Evaluation Rating = $\frac{\text{Points received}}{\text{Points possible}}$ = _____ = _____ %

INSTRUCTOR EVALUATION RATING

Five Views	Clearly Drawn	Accurate Sizing	General Features Included	Specific Features Included
1. Facial View				
2. Lingual View				
3. Mesial View				
4. Distal View				
5. Incisal/ Occlusal View				

Instructor Evaluation Rating = $\frac{\text{Points received}}{\text{Points possible}}$ = _____ = _____ %

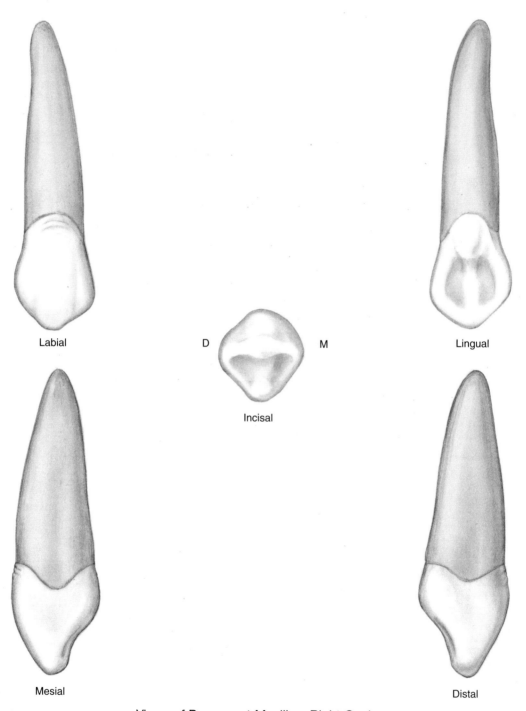

Labial

D   M

Incisal

Lingual

Mesial

Distal

Views of Permanent Maxillary Right Canine

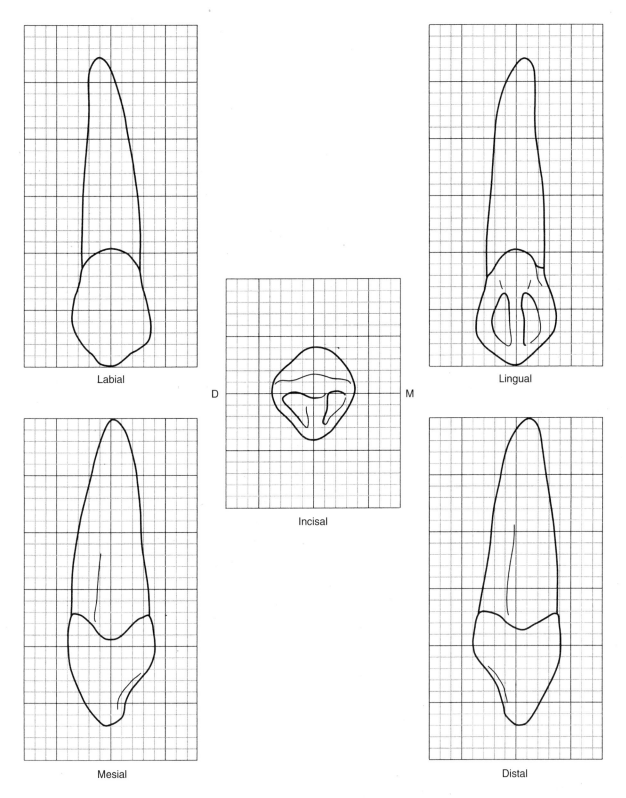

Labial

D

Incisal

M

Lingual

Mesial

Distal

Outline Views of a Permanent Maxillary Right Canine

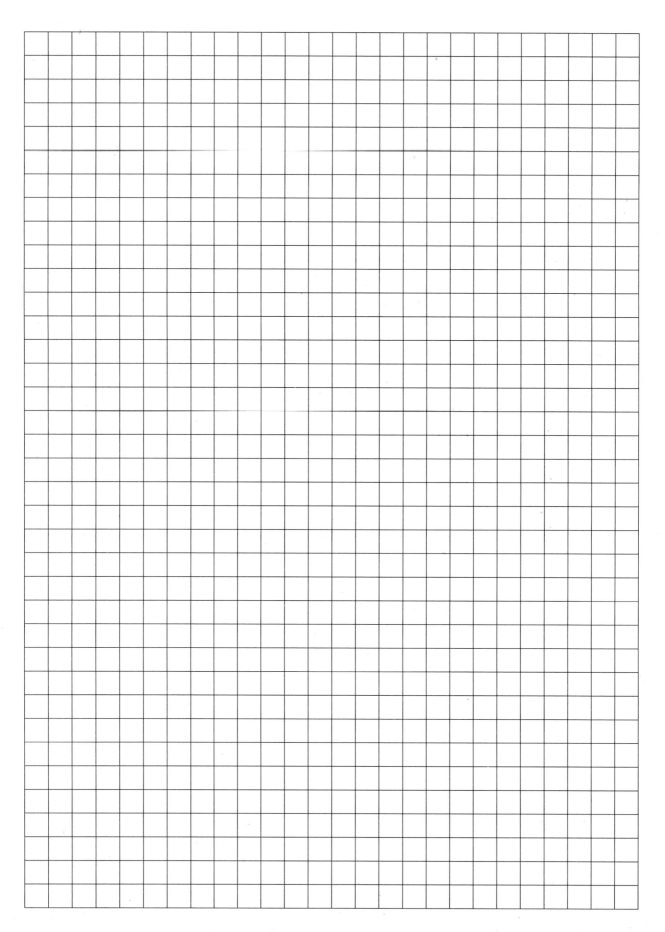

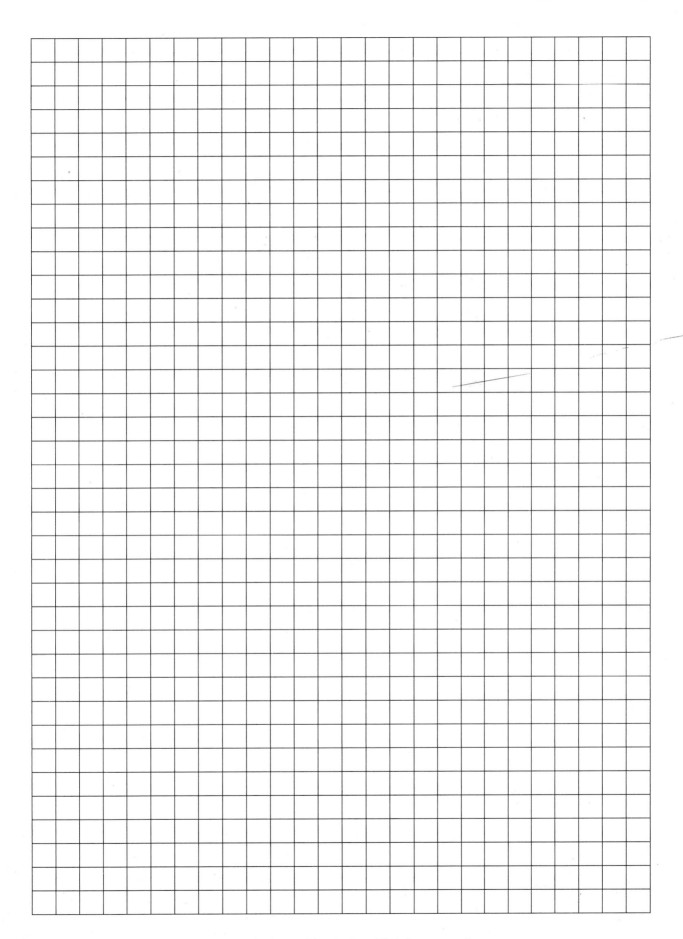

MEASUREMENTS FOR PERMANENT MAXILLARY CANINE*	
Cervico-Incisal Length of Crown	10.0
Length of Root	17.0
Mesiodistal Diameter of Crown	7.5
Mesiodistal Diameter of CEJ	5.5
Labiolingual Diameter	8.0
Labiolingual Diameter of CEJ	7.0
Curvature of CEJ at Mesial	2.5
Curvature of CEJ at Distal	1.5

*In millimeters; adapted from Nelson SJ: *Wheeler's Dental Anatomy, Physiology, and Occlusion.* 10th ed. Philadelphia: Elsevier; 2015.

CHECKLIST FOR PERMANENT MAXILLARY CANINE	
Features Noted	**Features Present**
Crown Features	
Single cusp with tip, slopes, labial ridge, cingulum, lingual ridge, marginal ridges, lingual fossae	
Prominent lingual surface with sharp cusp tip	
Shorter mesial cusp slope with more pronounced mesial CEJ curvature	
More cervical contact on distal	
Shorter distal outline on labial view with depression between distal contact and CEJ	
Height of contour for labial in cervical third and for lingual in middle third	
Mesial contact at junction of incisal third and middle thirds	
Distal contact at middle third	
Root Features	
Long thick single root	
Proximal root concavities and blunt root apex	

Name _____   Tooth Number/Name _____

Date _____   Instructor Rating _____

DRAWING EVALUATION CHECKLIST

RATING SCALE

Completely Correct = 2 points   Major Error = 0 points
Minor Error = 1 point   Note = NA (nonappropriate)

SELF-EVALUATION RATING

Five Views	Clearly Drawn	Accurate Sizing	General Features Included	Specific Features Included
1. Facial View				
2. Lingual View				
3. Mesial View				
4. Distal View				
5. Incisal/ Occlusal View				

$$\text{Self-Evaluation Rating} = \frac{\text{Points received}}{\text{Points possible}} = \underline{\hspace{2cm}} = \underline{\hspace{2cm}} \%$$

INSTRUCTOR EVALUATION RATING

Five Views	Clearly Drawn	Accurate Sizing	General Features Included	Specific Features Included
1. Facial View				
2. Lingual View				
3. Mesial View				
4. Distal View				
5. Incisal/ Occlusal View				

$$\text{Instructor Evaluation Rating} = \frac{\text{Points received}}{\text{Points possible}} = \underline{\hspace{2cm}} = \underline{\hspace{2cm}} \%$$

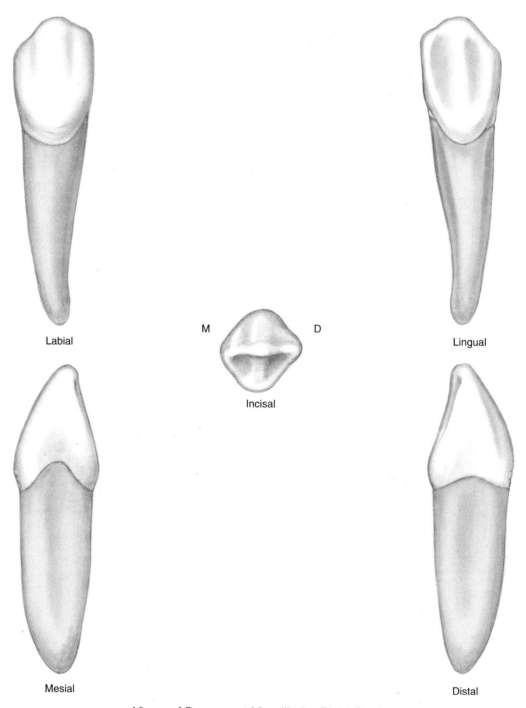

Labial

Lingual

M   D

Incisal

Mesial

Distal

Views of Permanent Mandibular Right Canine

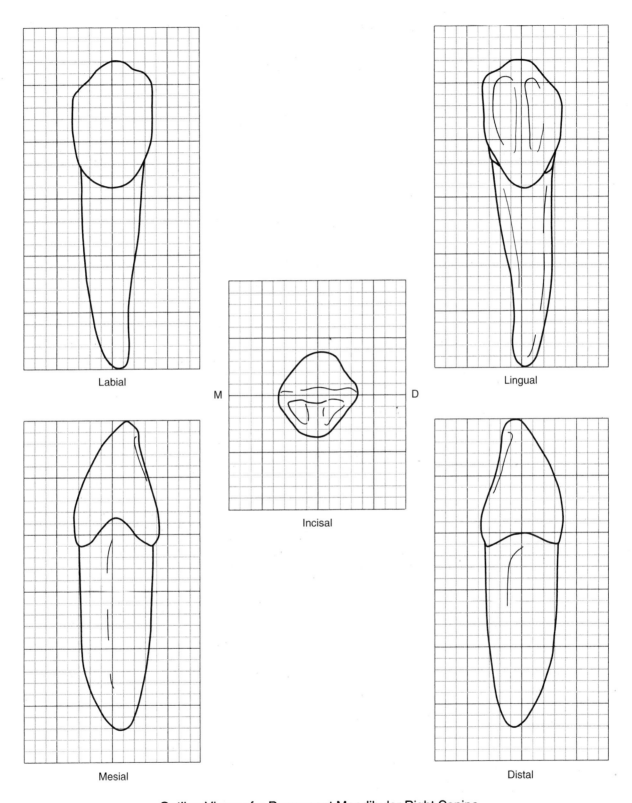

Labial

Lingual

M   D

Incisal

Mesial

Distal

Outline Views of a Permanent Mandibular Right Canine

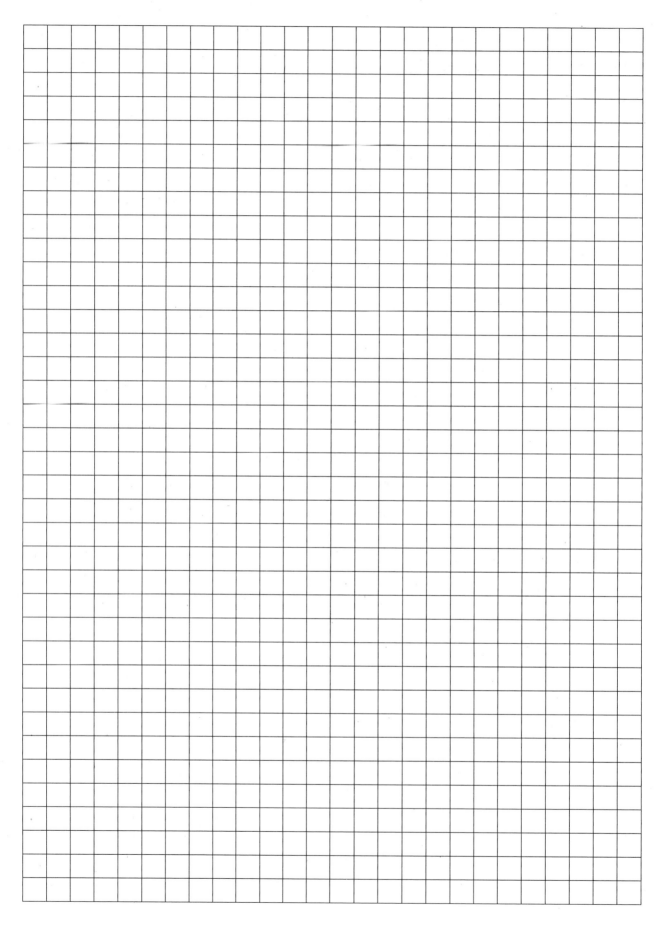

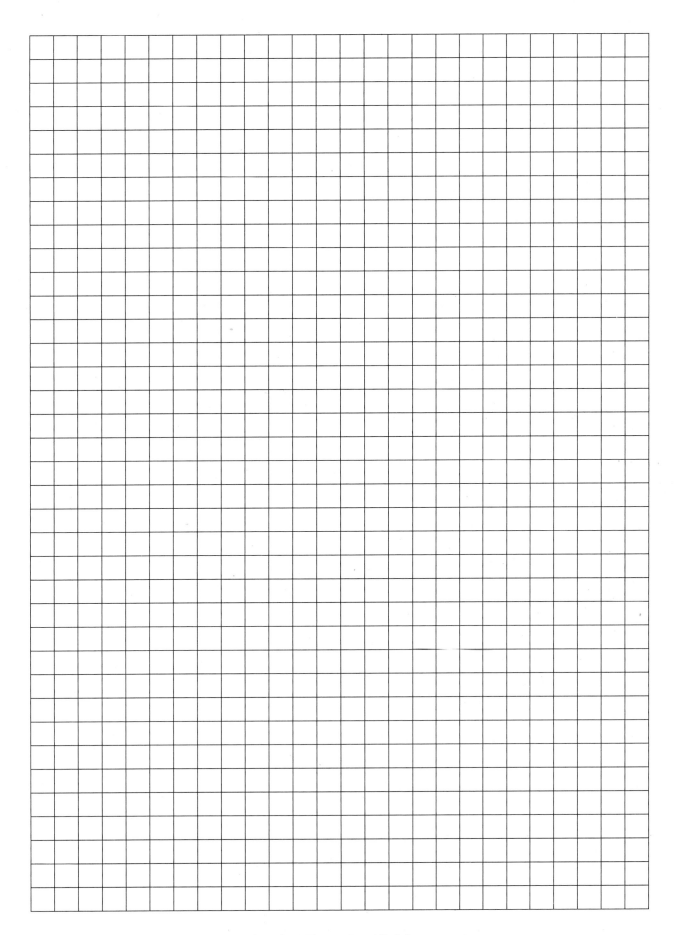

MEASUREMENTS FOR PERMANENT MANDIBULAR CANINE*	
Cervico-Incisal Length of Crown	11.0
Length of Root	16.0
Mesiodistal Diameter of Crown	7.0
Mesiodistal Diameter of CEJ	5.5
Labiolingual Diameter	7.5
Labiolingual Diameter of CEJ	7.0
Curvature of CEJ at Mesial	2.5
Curvature of CEJ at Distal	1.0

*In millimeters; adapted from Nelson SJ: *Wheeler's Dental Anatomy, Physiology, and Occlusion.* 10th ed. Philadelphia: Elsevier; 2015.

CHECKLIST FOR PERMANENT MANDIBULAR CANINE	
Features Noted	**Features Present**
Crown Features	
Single cusp with tip, slopes, labial ridge, cingulum, lingual ridge, marginal ridges, lingual fossae	
Less pronounced lingual surface with less sharp cusp tip	
Shorter mesial cusp slope with more pronounced mesial CEJ curvature	
More cervical contact on distal	
Shorter and rounder distal outline on labial view with shorter mesial slope than distal	
Height of contour for labial in cervical third and for lingual in middle third	
Mesial contact at incisal third	
Distal contact at junction of incisal and middle thirds	
Root Features	
Long thick single root	
Proximal root concavities with developmental depressions on mesial and distal giving tooth double-rooted appearance and pointed apex	

Name _____   Tooth Number/Name _____

Date _____ _____   Instructor Rating _____

DRAWING EVALUATION CHECKLIST

RATING SCALE
Completely Correct = 2 points   Major Error = 0 points
Minor Error = 1 point   Note = NA (nonappropriate)

SELF-EVALUATION RATING

Five Views	Clearly Drawn	Accurate Sizing	General Features Included	Specific Features Included
1. Facial View				
2. Lingual View				
3. Mesial View				
4. Distal View				
5. Incisal/ Occlusal View				

Self-Evaluation Rating = $\dfrac{\text{Points received}}{\text{Points possible}}$ = _____ = _____ %

INSTRUCTOR EVALUATION RATING

Five Views	Clearly Drawn	Accurate Sizing	General Features Included	Specific Features Included
1. Facial View				
2. Lingual View				
3. Mesial View				
4. Distal View				
5. Incisal/ Occlusal View				

Instructor Evaluation Rating = $\dfrac{\text{Points received}}{\text{Points possible}}$ = _____ = _____ %

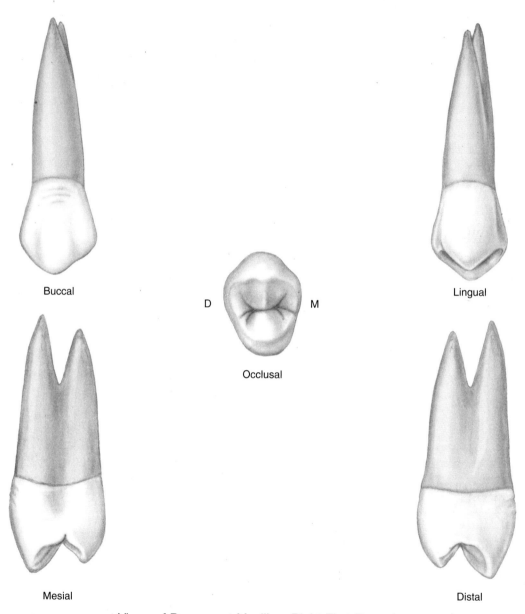

Buccal

D M

Occlusal

Lingual

Mesial

Distal

Views of Permanent Maxillary Right First Premolar

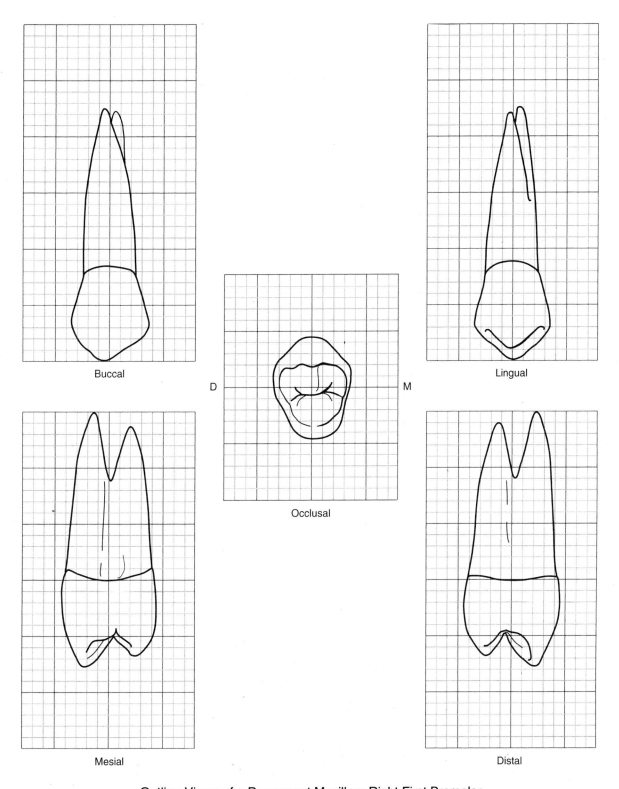

Buccal

Lingual

D

M

Occlusal

Mesial

Distal

Outline Views of a Permanent Maxillary Right First Premolar

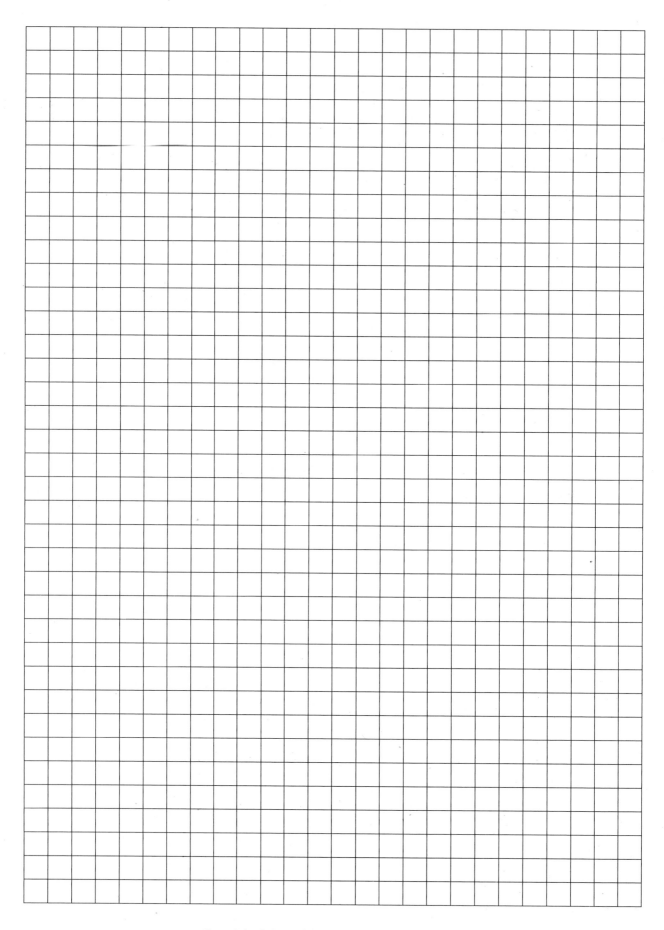

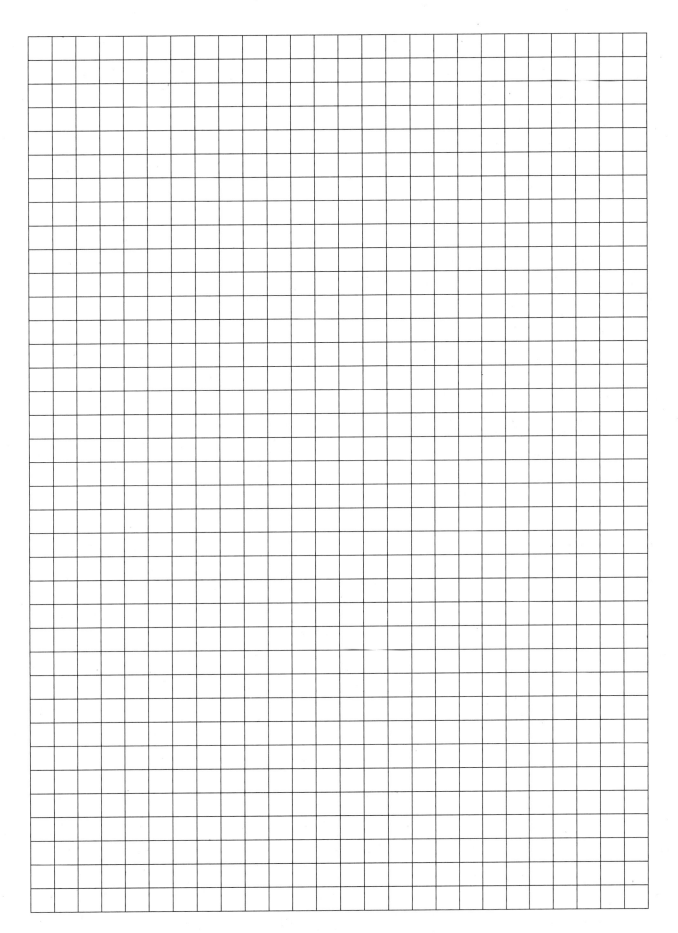

MEASUREMENTS FOR PERMANENT MAXILLARY FIRST PREMOLAR*

Cervico-Occlusal Length of Crown	8.5
Length of Root	14.0
Mesiodistal Diameter of Crown	7.0
Mesiodistal Diameter of CEJ	5.0
Buccolingual Diameter	9.0
Buccolingual Diameter of CEJ	8.0
Curvature of CEJ at Mesial	1.0
Curvature of CEJ at Distal	0.0

*In millimeters; adapted from Nelson SJ: *Wheeler's Dental Anatomy, Physiology, and Occlusion.* 10th ed. Philadelphia: Elsevier; 2015.

CHECKLIST FOR PERMANENT MAXILLARY FIRST PREMOLAR

Features Noted	Features Present
Crown Features	
Occlusal table with marginal ridges and cusps with tips, ridges, inclined planes, grooves	
Buccal cusp longer of two cusps with long central groove	
Longer mesial cusp slope than distal cusp slope and with mesial features: deeper CEJ curvature, marginal groove, developmental depression	
Buccal ridge	
Height of contour for buccal in cervical third and lingual in middle third	
Mesial and distal contact just cervical to junction of occlusal and middle thirds	
Root Features	
Two roots with root trunk	
Proximal root concavities	

Name _____   Tooth Number/Name _____

Date _____   Instructor Rating _____

DRAWING EVALUATION CHECKLIST

RATING SCALE

Completely Correct = 2 points   Major Error = 0 points
Minor Error = 1 point   Note = NA (nonappropriate)

SELF-EVALUATION RATING

Five Views	Clearly Drawn	Accurate Sizing	General Features Included	Specific Features Included
1. Facial View				
2. Lingual View				
3. Mesial View				
4. Distal View				
5. Incisal/ Occlusal View				

$$\text{Self-Evaluation Rating} = \frac{\text{Points received}}{\text{Points possible}} = \underline{\hspace{2cm}} = \underline{\hspace{2cm}} \%$$

INSTRUCTOR EVALUATION RATING

Five Views	Clearly Drawn	Accurate Sizing	General Features Included	Specific Features Included
1. Facial View				
2. Lingual View				
3. Mesial View				
4. Distal View				
5. Incisal/ Occlusal View				

$$\text{Instructor Evaluation Rating} = \frac{\text{Points received}}{\text{Points possible}} = \underline{\hspace{2cm}} = \underline{\hspace{2cm}} \%$$

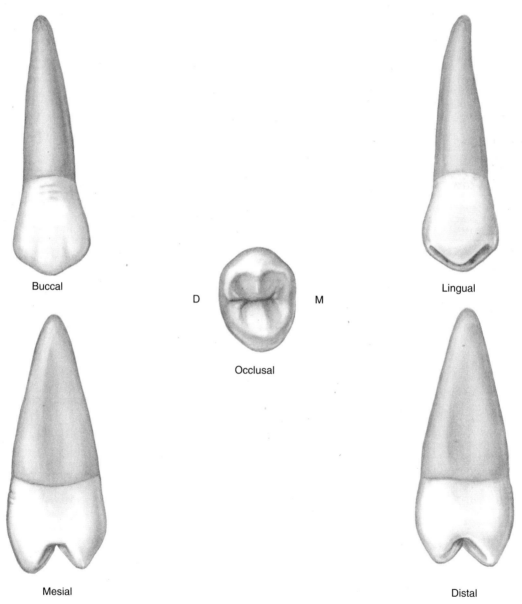

Buccal

Lingual

D   M

Occlusal

Mesial

Distal

View of Permanent Maxillary Right Second Premolar

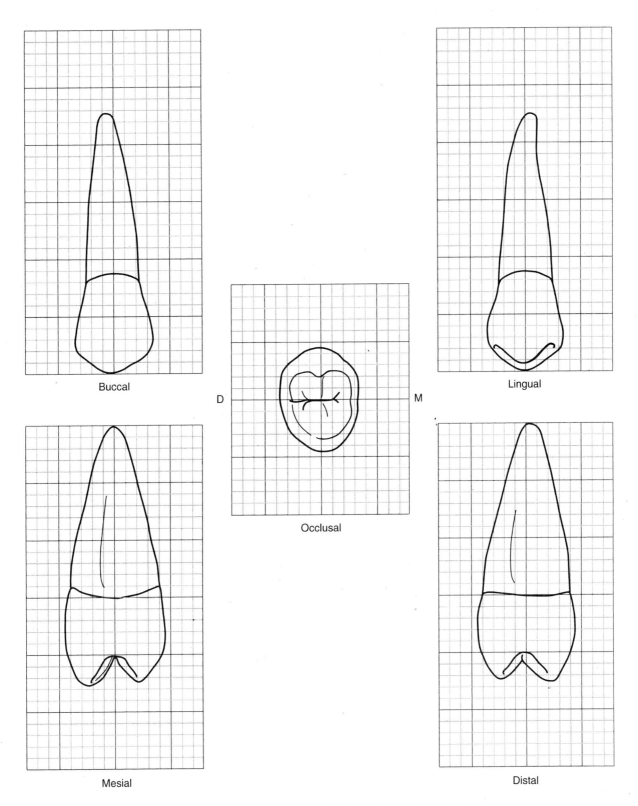

Buccal

Lingual

D ⎯ Occlusal ⎯ M

Mesial

Distal

Outline Views of a Permanent Maxillary Right Second Premolar

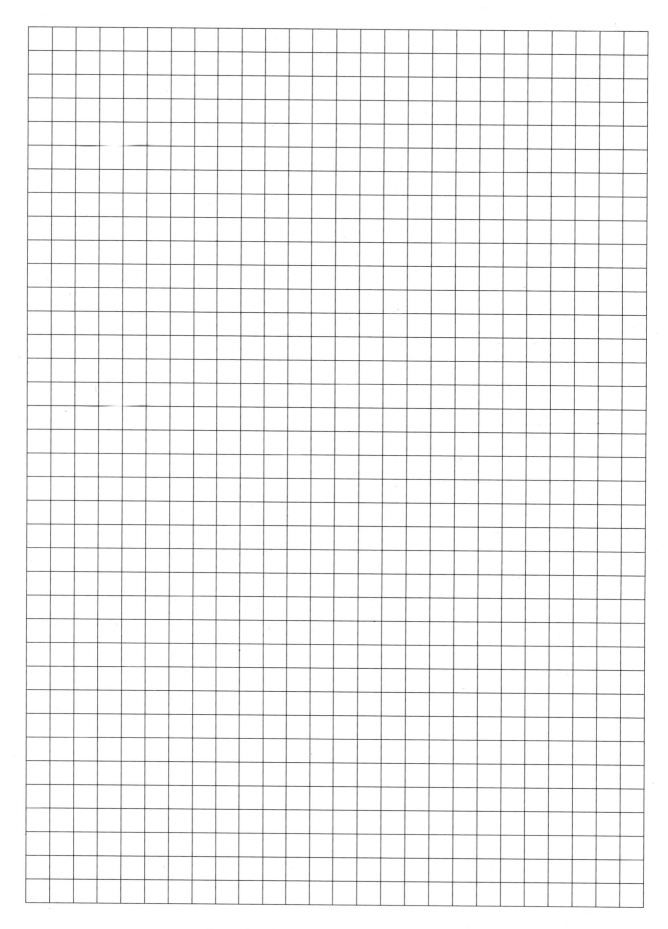

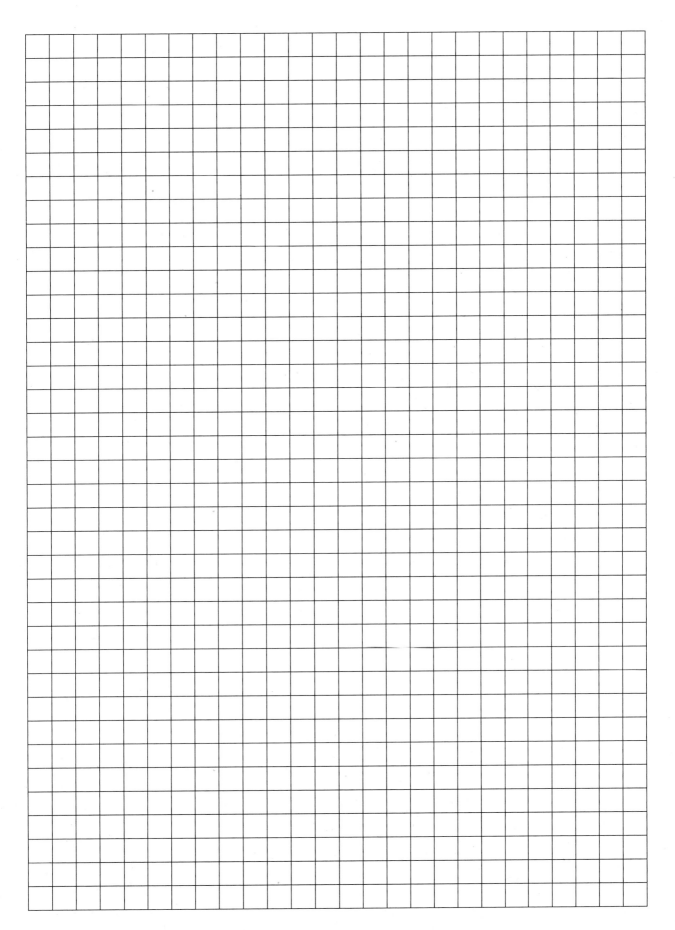

MEASUREMENTS FOR PERMANENT MAXILLARY SECOND PREMOLAR*

Cervico-Occlusal Length of Crown	8.5
Length of Root	14.0
Mesiodistal Diameter of Crown	7.0
Mesiodistal Diameter of CEJ	5.0
Buccolingual Diameter	9.0
Buccolingual Diameter of CEJ	8.0
Curvature of CEJ at Mesial	1.0
Curvature of CEJ at Distal	0.0

*In millimeters; adapted from Nelson SJ: *Wheeler's Dental Anatomy, Physiology, and Occlusion*. 10th ed. Philadelphia: Elsevier; 2015.

CHECKLIST FOR PERMANENT MAXILLARY SECOND PREMOLAR

Features Noted	Features Present
Crown Features	
Occlusal table with marginal ridges and cusps with tips, ridges, inclined planes, grooves fossae, pits	
Two cusps same length with short central groove	
Lingual cusp offset to the mesial	
Buccal ridge	
Height of contour for buccal in cervical third and lingual in middle third	
Mesial and distal contact just cervical to junction of occlusal and middle thirds	
Root Features	
Single rooted	
Proximal root concavities	

Name _____   Tooth Number/Name _____

Date _____   Instructor Rating _____

DRAWING EVALUATION CHECKLIST

RATING SCALE

Completely Correct = 2 points   Major Error = 0 points
Minor Error = 1 point   Note = NA (nonappropriate)

SELF-EVALUATION RATING

Five Views	Clearly Drawn	Accurate Sizing	General Features Included	Specific Features Included
1. Facial View				
2. Lingual View				
3. Mesial View				
4. Distal View				
5. Incisal/ Occlusal View				

Self-Evaluation Rating $= \dfrac{\text{Points received}}{\text{Points possible}} = $ _____ $= $ _____ %

INSTRUCTOR EVALUATION RATING

Five Views	Clearly Drawn	Accurate Sizing	General Features Included	Specific Features Included
1. Facial View				
2. Lingual View				
3. Mesial View				
4. Distal View				
5. Incisal/ Occlusal View				

Instructor Evaluation Rating $= \dfrac{\text{Points received}}{\text{Points possible}} = $ _____ $= $ _____ %

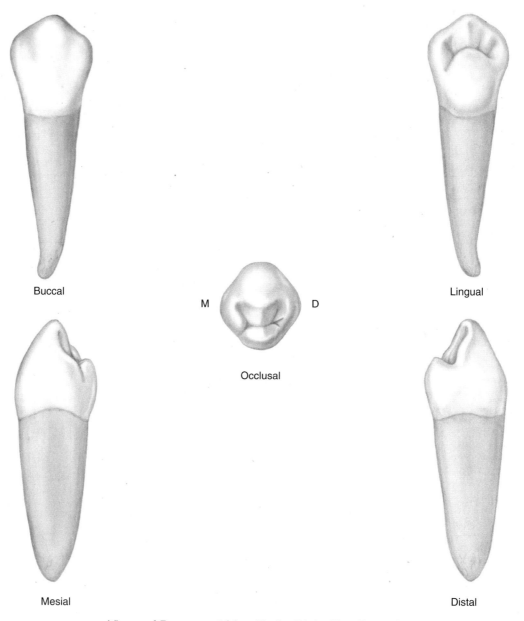

Buccal

Lingual

M   D

Occlusal

Mesial

Distal

Views of Permanent Mandibular Right First Premolar

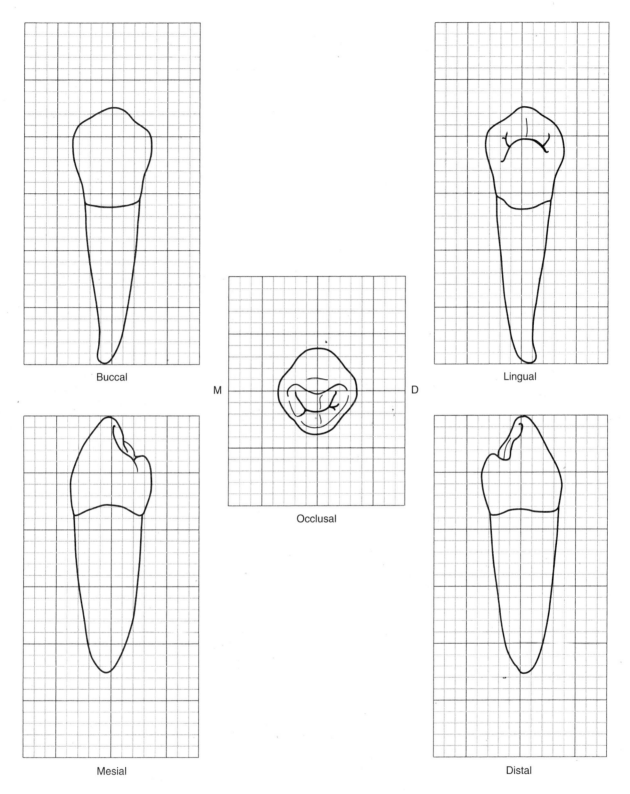

Buccal

Lingual

M   D

Occlusal

Mesial

Distal

Outline Views of a Permanent Mandibular Right First Premolar

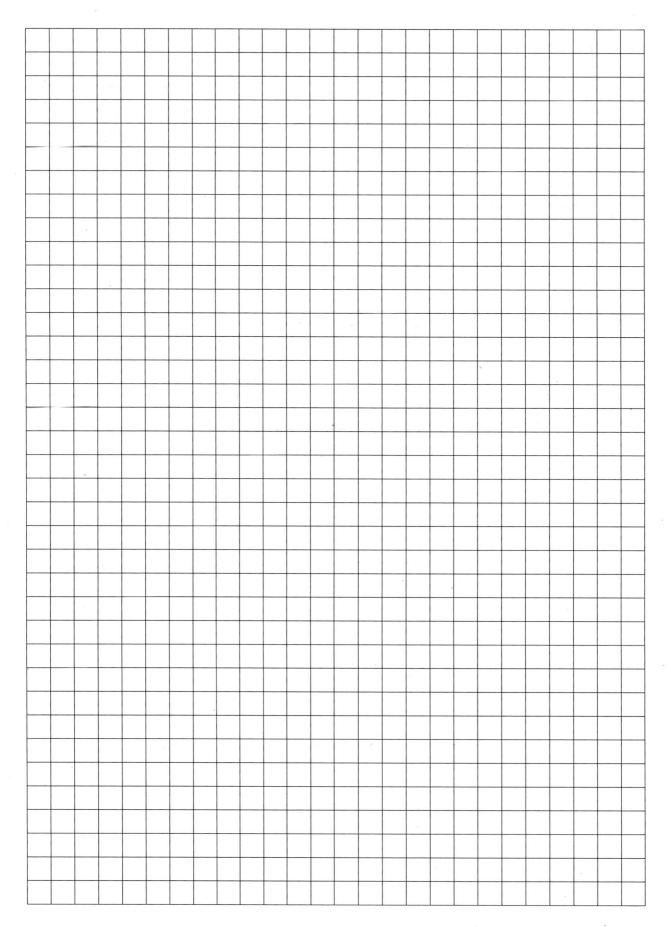

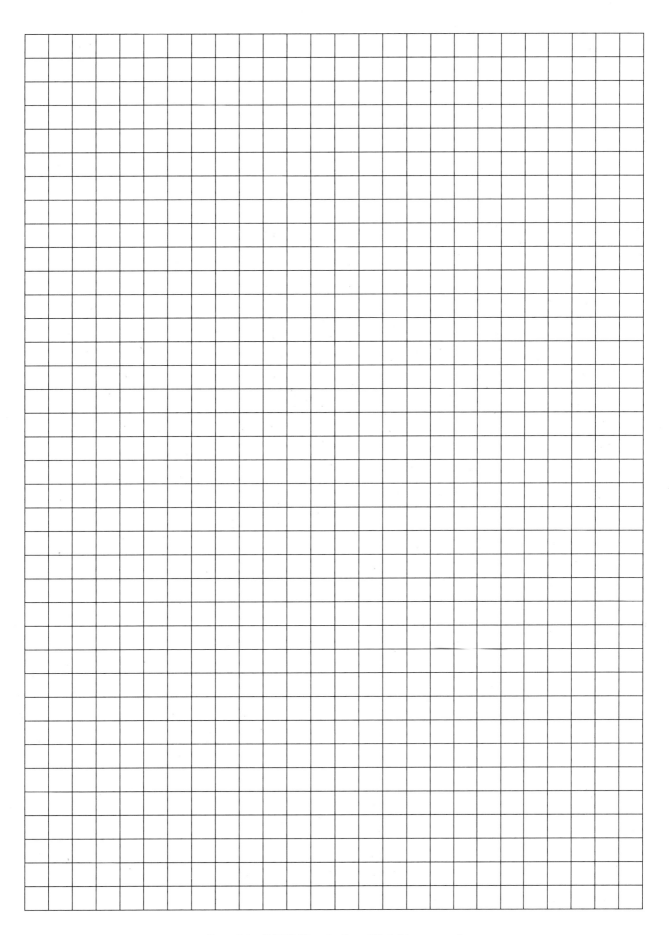

MEASUREMENTS FOR PERMANENT MANDIBULAR FIRST PREMOLAR*

Cervico-Occlusal Length of Crown	8.5
Length of Root	14.0
Mesiodistal Diameter of Crown	7.0
Mesiodistal Diameter of CEJ	5.0
Buccolingual Diameter	7.5
Buccolingual Diameter of CEJ	6.5
Curvature of CEJ at Mesial	1.0
Curvature of CEJ at Distal	0.0

*In millimeters; adapted from Nelson SJ: *Wheeler's Dental Anatomy, Physiology, and Occlusion*. 10th ed. Philadelphia: Elsevier; 2015.

CHECKLIST FOR PERMANENT MANDIBULAR FIRST PREMOLAR

Features Noted	Features Present
Crown Features	
Occlusal table with marginal ridges and cusps with tips, ridges, inclined planes, grooves, fossae, pits	
Smaller lingual cusp of two cusps	
Shorter mesial cusp slope with mesial surface features of deeper mesial CEJ curvature and mesiolingual groove	
Buccal ridge	
Height of contour for buccal in cervical third and lingual in middle third	
Mesial and distal contact just cervical to junction of occlusal and middle thirds	
Root Features	
Single rooted	
Proximal root concavities	

Name _____   Tooth Number/Name _____

Date _____   Instructor Rating _____

DRAWING EVALUATION CHECKLIST

RATING SCALE

Completely Correct = 2 points   Major Error = 0 points
Minor Error = 1 point   Note = NA (nonappropriate)

SELF-EVALUATION RATING

Five Views	Clearly Drawn	Accurate Sizing	General Features Included	Specific Features Included
1. Facial View				
2. Lingual View				
3. Mesial View				
4. Distal View				
5. Incisal/ Occlusal View				

Self-Evaluation Rating $= \dfrac{\text{Points received}}{\text{Points possible}} =$ _____ $=$ _____ %

INSTRUCTOR EVALUATION RATING

Five Views	Clearly Drawn	Accurate Sizing	General Features Included	Specific Features Included
1. Facial View				
2. Lingual View				
3. Mesial View				
4. Distal View				
5. Incisal/ Occlusal View				

Instructor Evaluation Rating $= \dfrac{\text{Points received}}{\text{Points possible}} =$ _____ $=$ _____ %

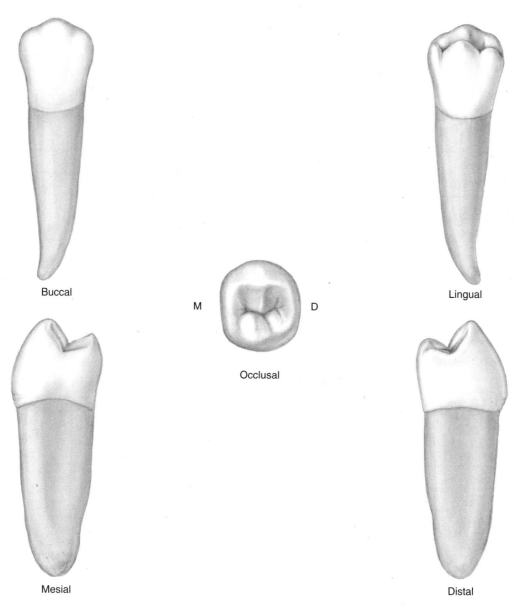

Buccal

Lingual

M

D

Occlusal

Mesial

Distal

Views of Permanent Mandibular Right Second Premolar (Three-Cusp Type)

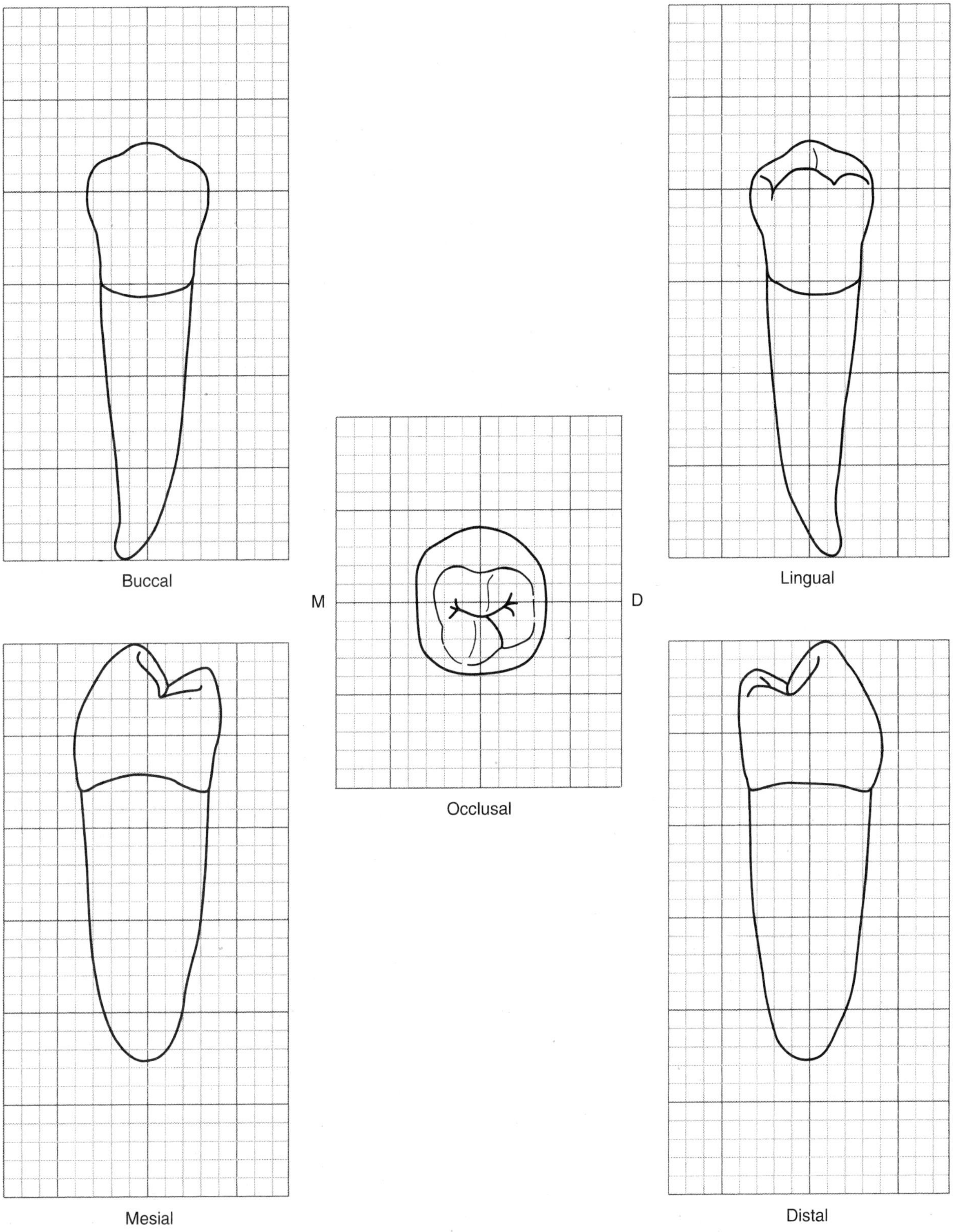

Buccal

M

D

Lingual

Occlusal

Mesial

Distal

Outline Views of Permanent Mandibular Right Second Premolar (Three-Cusp Type)

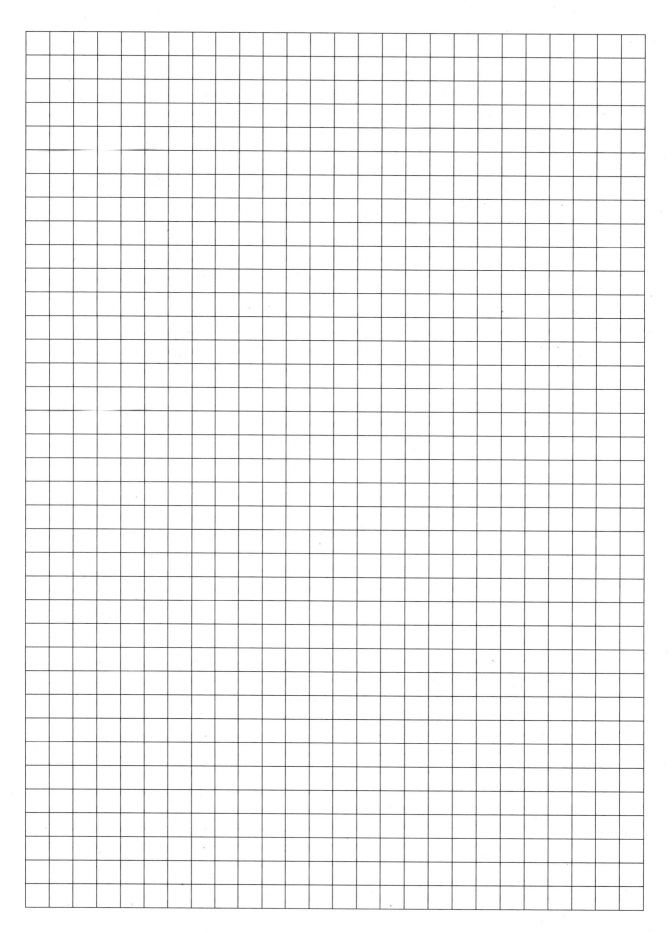

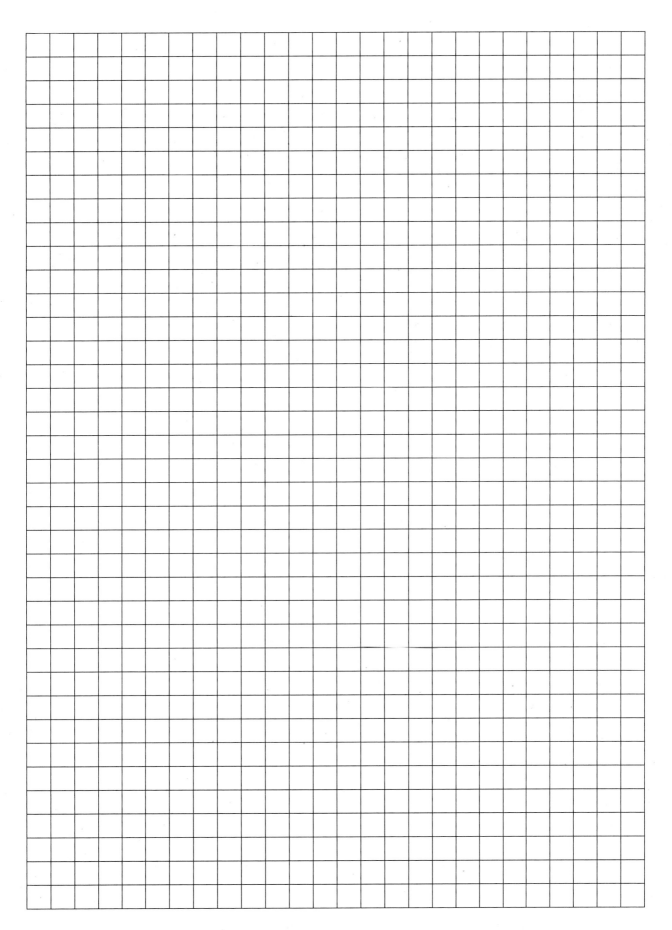

MEASUREMENTS FOR PERMANENT MANDIBULAR SECOND PREMOLAR (Three-Cusp Type)*	
Cervico-Occlusal Length of Crown	8.0
Length of Root	14.5
Mesiodistal Diameter of Crown	7.0
Mesiodistal Diameter of CEJ	5.0
Buccolingual Diameter	8.0
Buccolingual Diameter of CEJ	7.0
Curvature of CEJ at Mesial	1.0
Curvature of CEJ at Distal	0.0

*In millimeters; adapted from Nelson SJ: *Wheeler's Dental Anatomy, Physiology, and Occlusion.* 10th ed. Philadelphia: Elsevier; 2015.

CHECKLIST FOR PERMANENT MANDIBULAR SECOND PREMOLAR (Three-Cusp Type)	
Features Noted	**Features Present**
Crown Features	
Occlusal table with marginal ridges and cusps with tips, ridges, inclined planes, grooves	
Three cusps with Y-shaped groove pattern	
Distal marginal ridge more cervically located with more occlusal surface visible from distal view	
Buccal ridge	
Height of contour for buccal in cervical third and lingual in middle third	
Mesial and distal contact just cervical to junction of occlusal and middle thirds	
Root Features	
Single rooted	
Proximal root concavities	

Name _____ Tooth Number/Name _____

Date _____ Instructor Rating _____

DRAWING EVALUATION CHECKLIST

RATING SCALE
Completely Correct = 2 points   Major Error = 0 points
Minor Error = 1 point   Note = NA (nonappropriate)

SELF-EVALUATION RATING

Five Views	Clearly Drawn	Accurate Sizing	General Features Included	Specific Features Included
1. Facial View				
2. Lingual View				
3. Mesial View				
4. Distal View				
5. Incisal/ Occlusal View				

$$\text{Self-Evaluation Rating} = \frac{\text{Points received}}{\text{Points possible}} = \underline{\hspace{2cm}} = \underline{\hspace{2cm}} \%$$

INSTRUCTOR EVALUATION RATING

Five Views	Clearly Drawn	Accurate Sizing	General Features Included	Specific Features Included
1. Facial View				
2. Lingual View				
3. Mesial View				
4. Distal View				
5. Incisal/ Occlusal View				

$$\text{Instructor Evaluation Rating} = \frac{\text{Points received}}{\text{Points possible}} = \underline{\hspace{2cm}} = \underline{\hspace{2cm}} \%$$

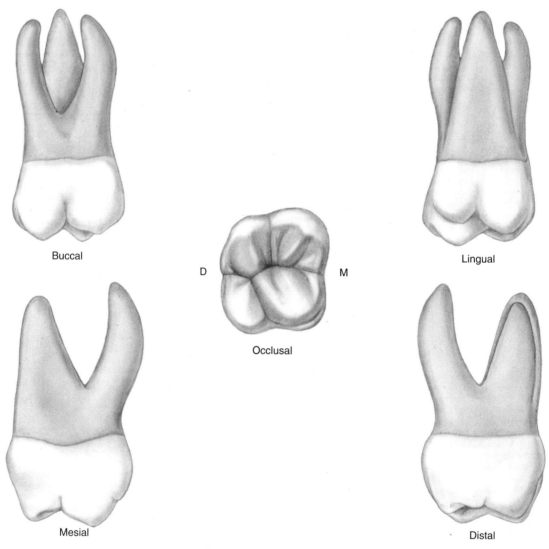

Buccal

Lingual

D   M

Occlusal

Mesial

Distal

Views of Permanent Maxillary Right First Molar

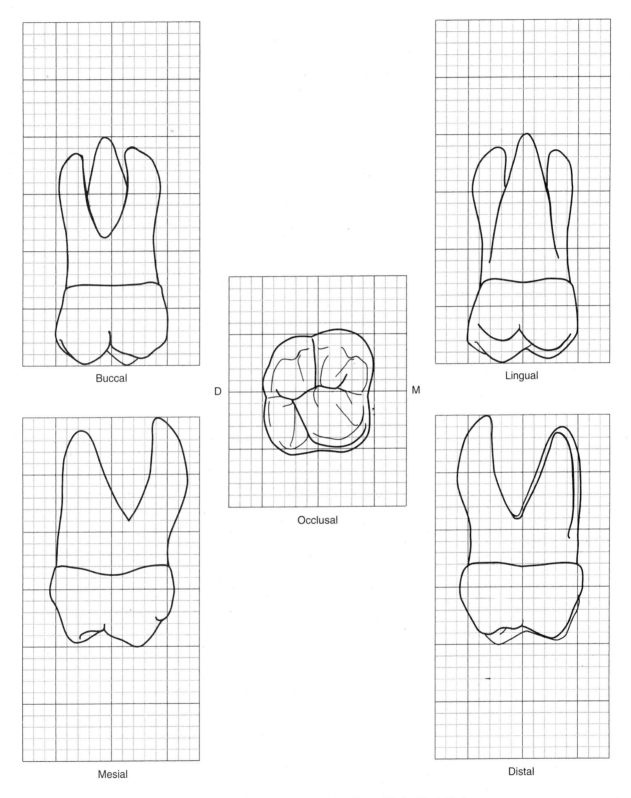

Buccal

Lingual

D   M

Occlusal

Mesial

Distal

Outline Views of a Permanent Maxillary Right First Molar

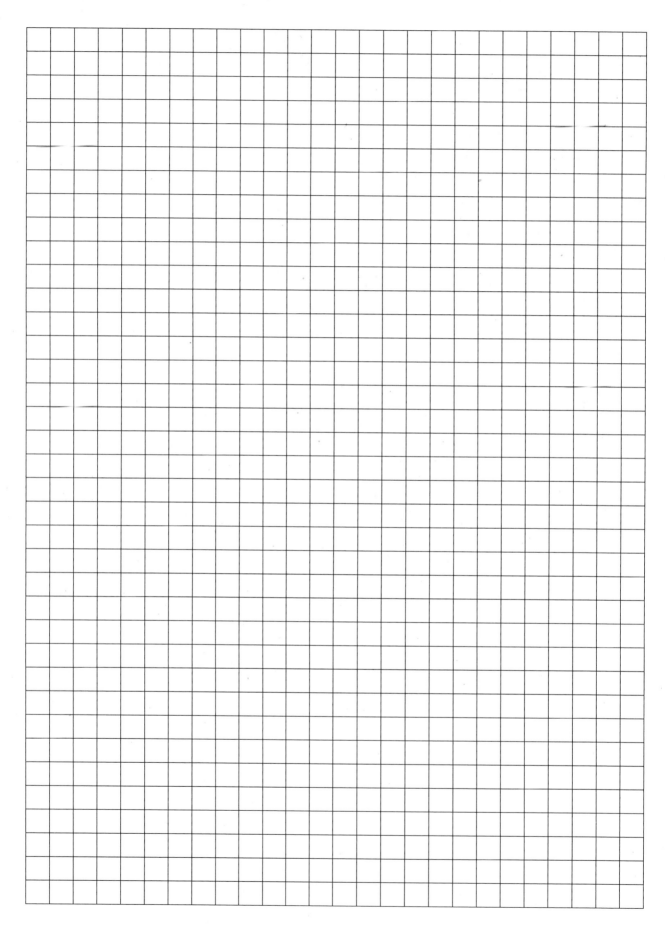

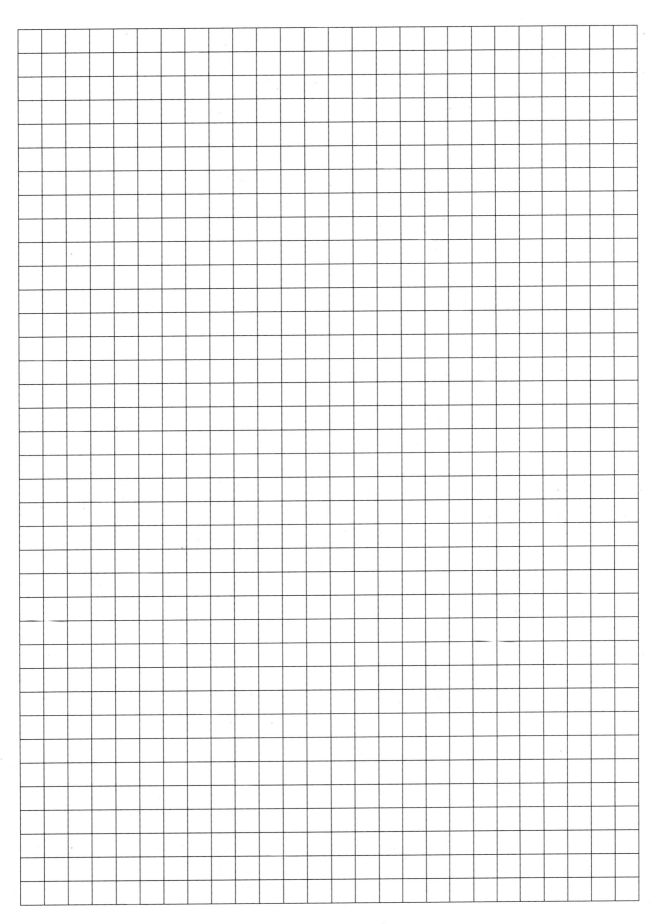

MEASUREMENTS FOR PERMANENT MAXILLARY FIRST MOLAR*

Cervico-Occlusal Length of Crown	7.5
Length of Root	Buccal: 12 Lingual: 13
Mesiodistal Diameter of Crown	10.0
Mesiodistal Diameter of CEJ	8.0
Buccolingual Diameter	11.0
Buccolingual Diameter of CEJ	10.0
Curvature of CEJ at Mesial	1.0
Curvature of CEJ at Distal	0.0

*In millimeters; adapted from Nelson SJ: *Wheeler's Dental Anatomy, Physiology, and Occlusion.* 10th ed. Philadelphia: Elsevier; 2015.

CHECKLIST FOR PERMANENT MAXILLARY FIRST MOLAR

Features Noted	Features Present
Crown Features	
Occlusal table with marginal ridges and cusps with tips, ridges, inclined planes, grooves, fossae, pits	
Prominent oblique ridge	
Four major cusps with buccal cusps almost equal in height	
Fifth minor cusp of Carabelli associated with mesiolingual cusp and groove	
Mesiolingual cusp outline longer and larger but not as sharp as distolingual cusp outline	
Buccal cervical ridge	
Height of contour for buccal in cervical third and lingual in middle third	
Mesial contact at junction of occlusal and middle thirds	
Distal contact at middle third	
Root Features	
Three roots	
Furcations well removed from CEJ, root trunks, root concavities, divergent roots	

Name _____   Tooth Number/Name _____
Date _____   Instructor Rating _____

DRAWING EVALUATION CHECKLIST

RATING SCALE

Completely Correct = 2 points   Major Error = 0 points
Minor Error = 1 point   Note = NA (nonappropriate)

SELF-EVALUATION RATING

Five Views	Clearly Drawn	Accurate Sizing	General Features Included	Specific Features Included
1. Facial View				
2. Lingual View				
3. Mesial View				
4. Distal View				
5. Incisal/ Occlusal View				

Self-Evaluation Rating = $\dfrac{\text{Points received}}{\text{Points possible}}$ = _____ = _____ %

INSTRUCTOR EVALUATION RATING

Five Views	Clearly Drawn	Accurate Sizing	General Features Included	Specific Features Included
1. Facial View				
2. Lingual View				
3. Mesial View				
4. Distal View				
5. Incisal/ Occlusal View				

Instructor Evaluation Rating = $\dfrac{\text{Points received}}{\text{Points possible}}$ = _____ = _____ %

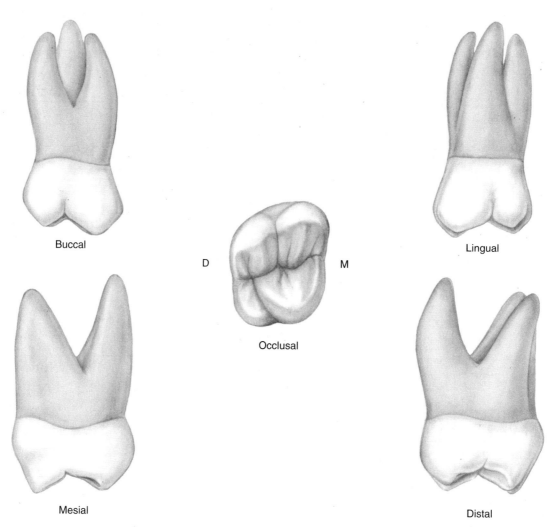

Buccal

Lingual

D　　　　M

Occlusal

Mesial

Distal

Views of Permanent Maxillary Right Second Molar (Rhomboidal Crown Outline)

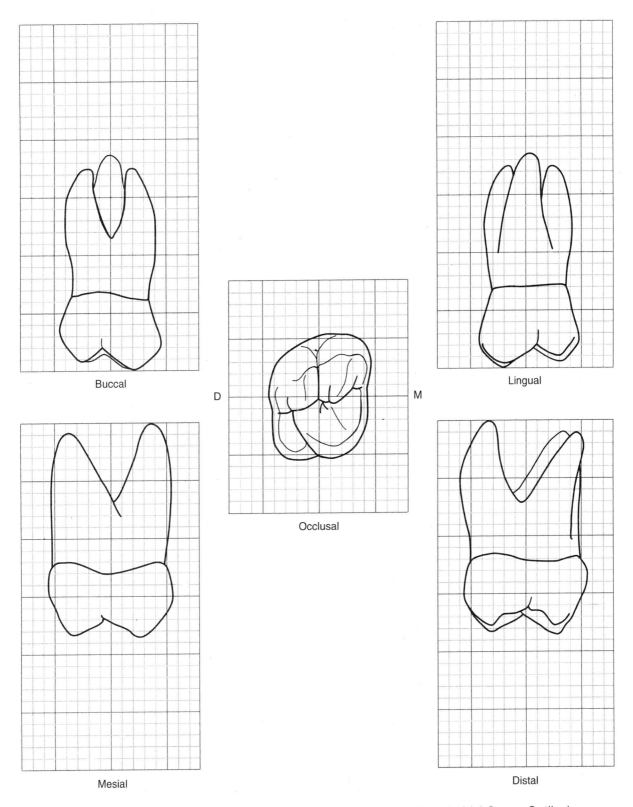

Buccal

Lingual

D   M

Occlusal

Mesial

Distal

Outline Views of Permanent Maxillary Right Second Molar (Rhomboidal Crown Outline)

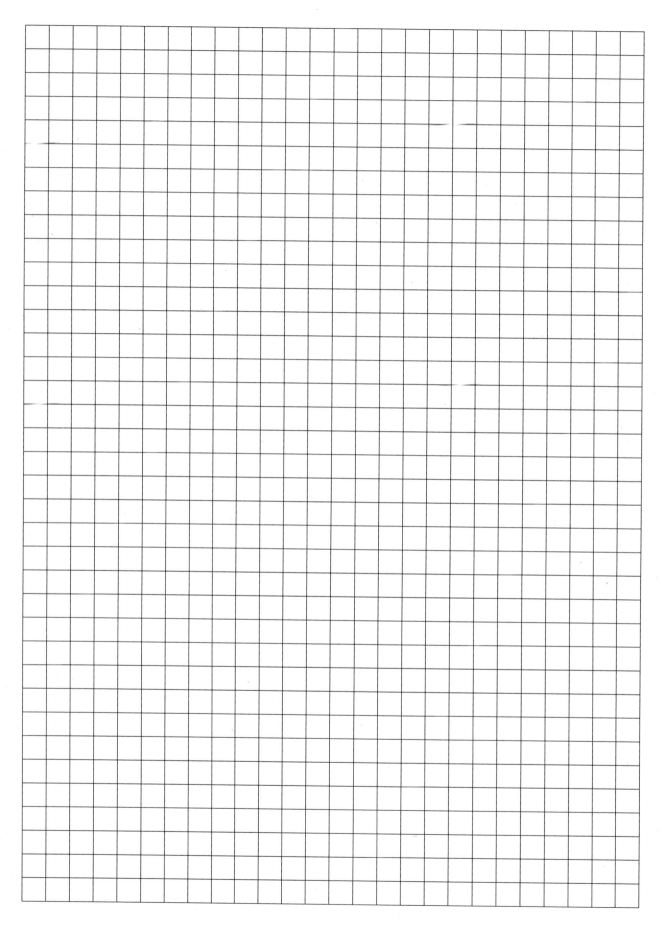

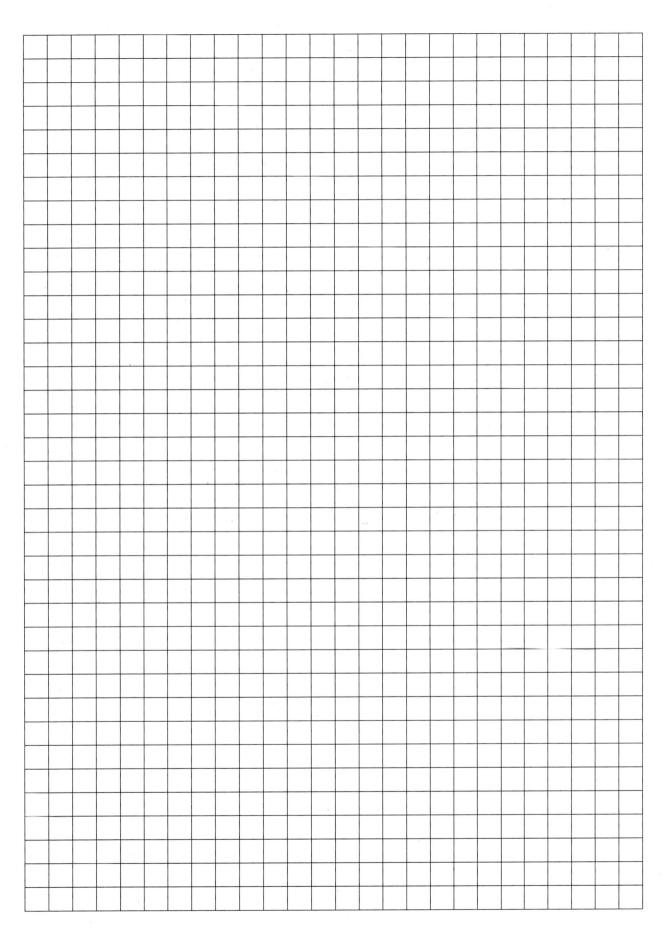

MEASUREMENTS FOR PERMANENT MAXILLARY SECOND MOLAR
(Rhomboidal Crown Outline)*

Cervico-Occlusal Length of Crown	7.0
Length of Root	Buccal: 11 Lingual: 12
Mesiodistal Diameter of Crown	9.0
Mesiodistal Diameter of CEJ	7.0
Buccolingual Diameter	11.0
Buccolingual Diameter of CEJ	10.0
Curvature of CEJ at Mesial	1.0
Curvature of CEJ at Distal	0.0

*In millimeters; adapted from Nelson SJ: *Wheeler's Dental Anatomy, Physiology, and Occlusion.* 10th ed. Philadelphia: Elsevier; 2015.

CHECKLIST FOR PERMANENT MAXILLARY SECOND MOLAR
(Rhomboidal Crown Outline)

Features Noted	Features Present
Crown Features	
Occlusal table with marginal ridges and cusps with tips, ridges, inclined planes, grooves, fossae, pits	
Less prominent oblique ridge	
Four cusps	
Mesiobuccal cusp longer than distobuccal cusp and distolingual cusp smaller	
Buccal cervical ridge	
Height of contour for buccal in cervical third and lingual in middle third	
Mesial contact at middle third	
Distal contact at middle third	
Root Features	
Three roots	
Furcations, root trunks, root concavities, less divergent roots	

Name _____   Tooth Number/Name _____

Date _____   Instructor Rating _____

DRAWING EVALUATION CHECKLIST

RATING SCALE

Completely Correct = 2 points   Major Error = 0 points
Minor Error = 1 point   Note = NA (nonappropriate)

SELF-EVALUATION RATING

Five Views	Clearly Drawn	Accurate Sizing	General Features Included	Specific Features Included
1. Facial View				
2. Lingual View				
3. Mesial View				
4. Distal View				
5. Incisal/ Occlusal View				

$$\text{Self-Evaluation Rating} = \frac{\text{Points received}}{\text{Points possible}} = \underline{\hspace{2cm}} = \underline{\hspace{2cm}} \%$$

INSTRUCTOR EVALUATION RATING

Five Views	Clearly Drawn	Accurate Sizing	General Features Included	Specific Features Included
1. Facial View				
2. Lingual View				
3. Mesial View				
4. Distal View				
5. Incisal/ Occlusal View				

$$\text{Instructor Evaluation Rating} = \frac{\text{Points received}}{\text{Points possible}} = \underline{\hspace{2cm}} = \underline{\hspace{2cm}} \%$$

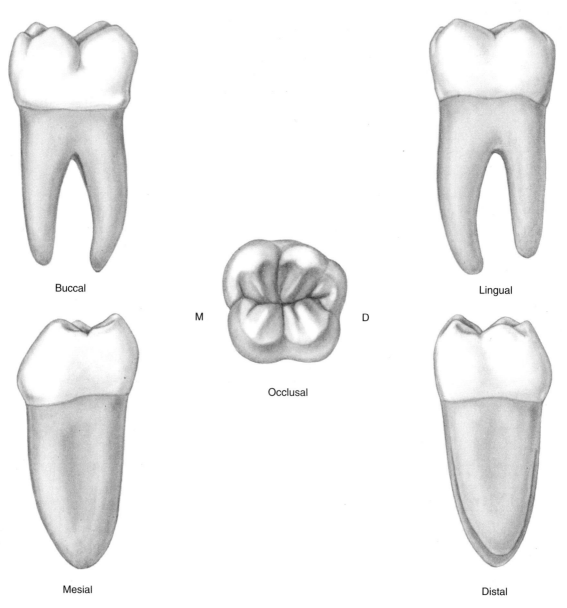

Buccal

Lingual

M   D

Occlusal

Mesial

Distal

Views of Permanent Mandibular Right First Molar

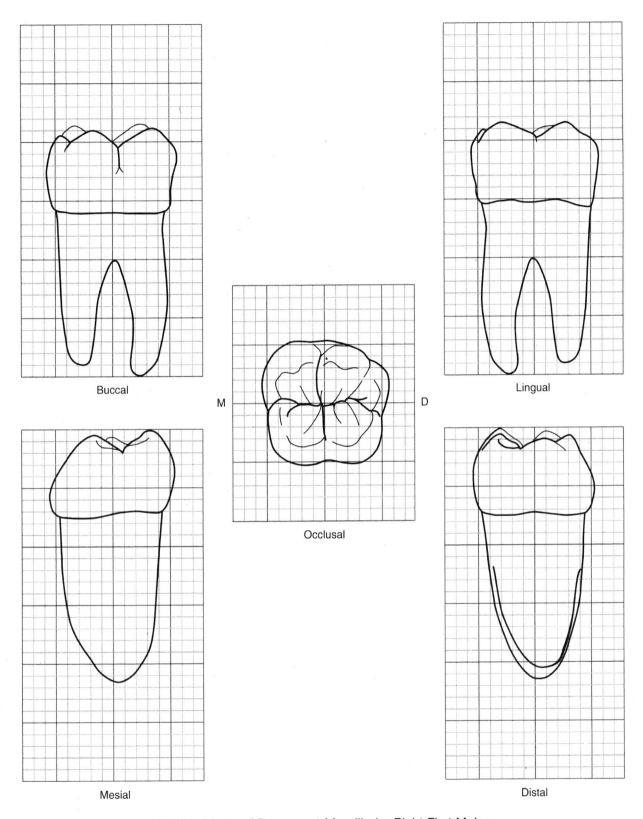

Buccal

Lingual

M

D

Occlusal

Mesial

Distal

Outline Views of Permanent Mandibular Right First Molar

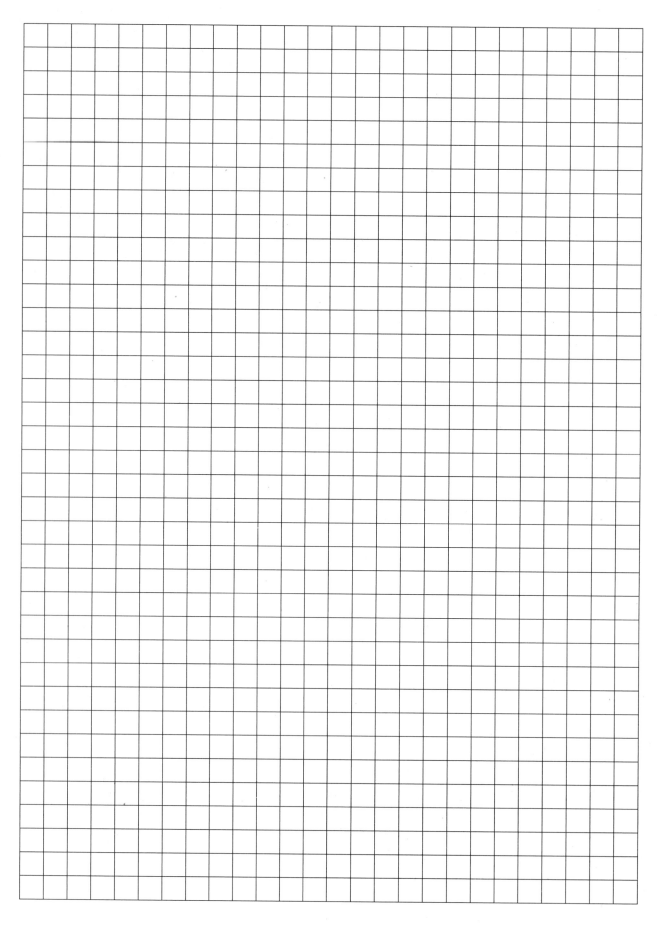

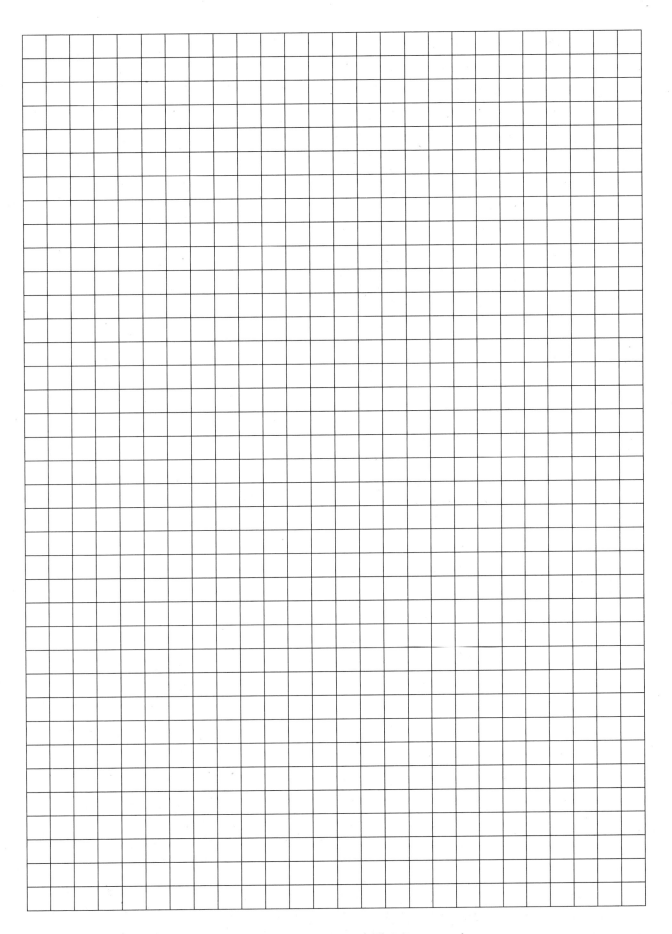

MEASUREMENTS FOR PERMANENT MANDIBULAR FIRST MOLAR*

Cervico-Occlusal Length of Crown	7.5
Length of Root	14.0
Mesiodistal Diameter of Crown	11.0
Mesiodistal Diameter of CEJ	9.0
Buccolingual Diameter	10.5
Buccolingual Diameter of CEJ	9.0
Curvature of CEJ at Mesial	1.0
Curvature of CEJ at Distal	0.0

*In millimeters; adapted from Nelson SJ: *Wheeler's Dental Anatomy, Physiology*, and Occlusion. 10th ed. Philadelphia: Elsevier; 2015.

CHECKLIST FOR PERMANENT MANDIBULAR FIRST MOLAR

Features Noted	Features Present
Crown Features	
Occlusal table with marginal ridges and cusps with tips, ridges, inclined planes, grooves, fossae, pits	
Five cusps with Y-shaped groove pattern and buccal groove	
Distal cusp smallest with sharp cusp	
Buccal cervical ridge	
Height of contour for buccal in cervical third and lingual in middle third	
Mesial and distal contact at junction of occlusal and middle thirds	
Root Features	
Two roots	
Furcations well removed from CEJ, root trunks, root concavities, divergent roots	

Name _____   Tooth Number/Name _____

Date _____   Instructor Rating _____

DRAWING EVALUATION CHECKLIST

RATING SCALE

Completely Correct = 2 points   Major Error = 0 points
Minor Error = 1 point   Note = NA (nonappropriate)

SELF-EVALUATION RATING

Five Views	Clearly Drawn	Accurate Sizing	General Features Included	Specific Features Included
1. Facial View				
2. Lingual View				
3. Mesial View				
4. Distal View				
5. Incisal/ Occlusal View				

Self-Evaluation Rating $= \dfrac{\text{Points received}}{\text{Points possible}} =$ _____ $=$ _____ %

INSTRUCTOR EVALUATION RATING

Five Views	Clearly Drawn	Accurate Sizing	General Features Included	Specific Features Included
1. Facial View				
2. Lingual View				
3. Mesial View				
4. Distal View				
5. Incisal/ Occlusal View				

Instructor Evaluation Rating $= \dfrac{\text{Points received}}{\text{Points possible}} =$ _____ $=$ _____ %

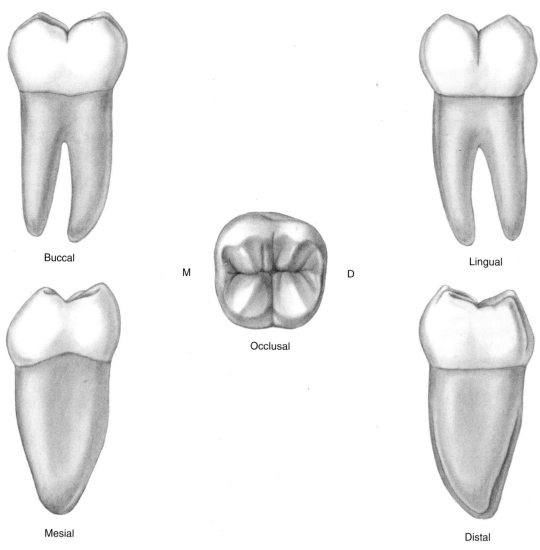

Buccal

Lingual

M   D

Occlusal

Mesial

Distal

Views of Permanent Mandibular Right Second Molar

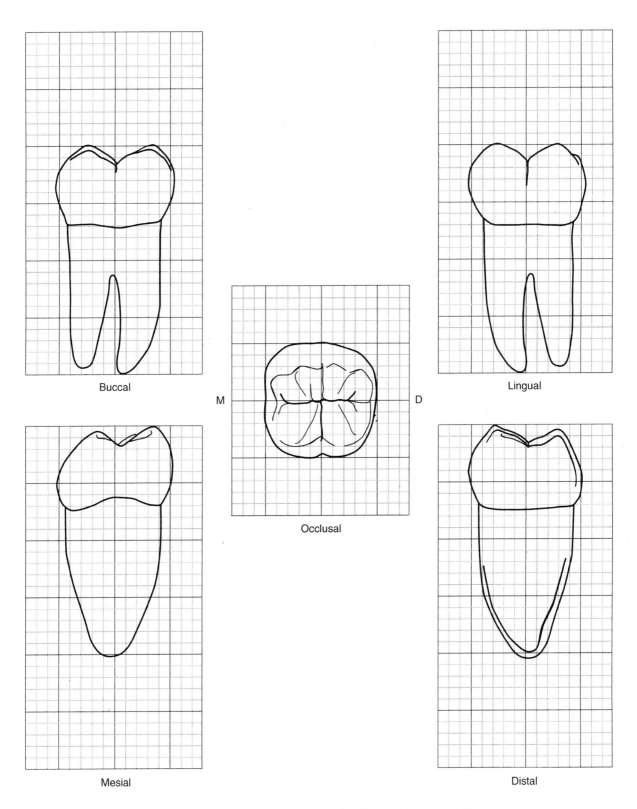

Buccal

Lingual

M   D

Occlusal

Mesial

Distal

Outline Views of Permanent Mandibular Right Second Molar

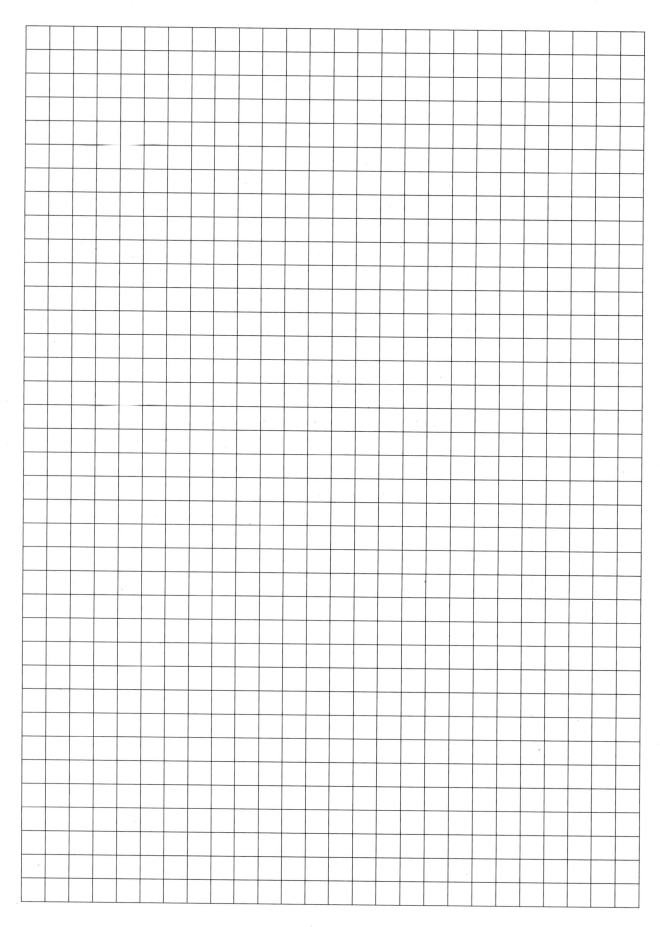

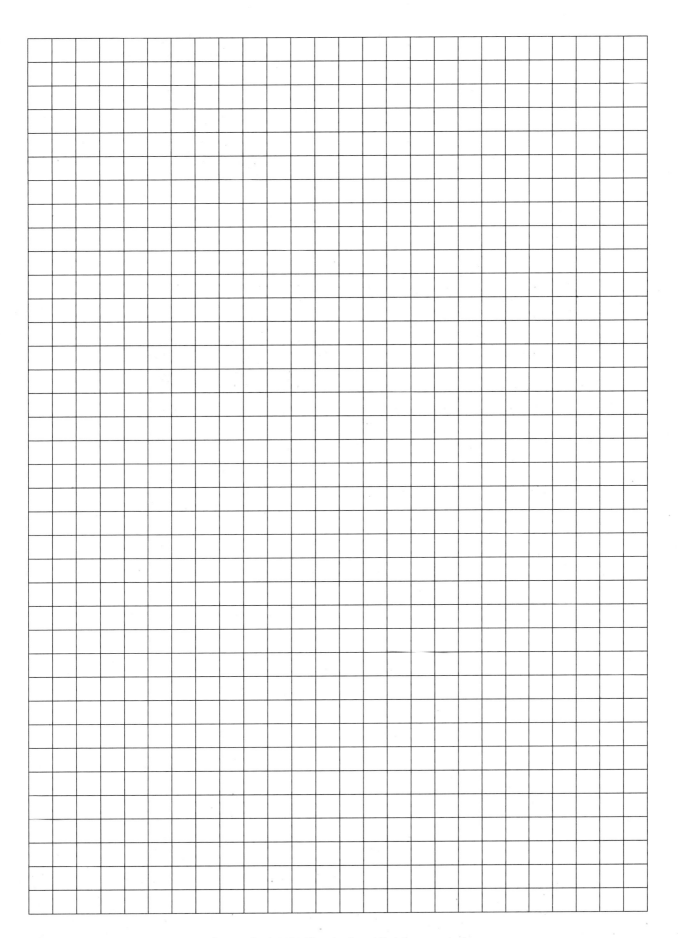

MEASUREMENTS FOR PERMANENT MANDIBULAR SECOND MOLAR*	
Cervico-Occlusal Length of Crown	7.0
Length of Root	13.0
Mesiodistal Diameter of Crown	10.5
Mesiodistal Diameter of CEJ	8.0
Buccolingual Diameter	10.0
Buccolingual Diameter of CEJ	9.0
Curvature of CEJ at Mesial	1.0
Curvature of CEJ at Distal	0.0

*In millimeters; adapted from Nelson SJ: *Wheeler's Dental Anatomy, Physiology, and Occlusion.* 10th ed. Philadelphia: Elsevier; 2015.

CHECKLIST FOR PERMANENT MANDIBULAR SECOND MOLAR	
Features Noted	**Features Present**
Crown Features	
Occlusal table with marginal ridges and cusps with tips, ridges, inclined planes, grooves, fossae, pits	
Four cusps with cross-shaped groove pattern	
Difference in height of contour for buccal and lingual from each proximal surface and wider on mesial than distal	
Buccal cervical ridge	
Height of contour for buccal in cervical third and lingual in middle third	
Mesial and distal contact at middle third	
Root Features	
Two roots	
Furcations closer to CEJ, root trunks, root concavities, less divergent roots	

Name _____   Tooth Number/Name _____

Date _____   Instructor Rating _____

DRAWING EVALUATION CHECKLIST

RATING SCALE

Completely Correct = 2 points   Major Error = 0 points
Minor Error = 1 point   Note = NA (nonappropriate)

SELF-EVALUATION RATING

Five Views	Clearly Drawn	Accurate Sizing	General Features Included	Specific Features Included
1. Facial View				
2. Lingual View				
3. Mesial View				
4. Distal View				
5. Incisal/ Occlusal View				

Self-Evaluation Rating = $\dfrac{\text{Points received}}{\text{Points possible}}$ = _____ = _____ %

INSTRUCTOR EVALUATION RATING

Five Views	Clearly Drawn	Accurate Sizing	General Features Included	Specific Features Included
1. Facial View				
2. Lingual View				
3. Mesial View				
4. Distal View				
5. Incisal/ Occlusal View				

Instructor Evaluation Rating = $\dfrac{\text{Points received}}{\text{Points possible}}$ = _____ = _____ %

General Recommendations

When studying dental anatomy, examining extracted teeth is a valuable supplement to studying the "ideal" form noted in plastic or plaster teeth. Extracted teeth provide a more realistic concept of the anatomy of the tooth because they have more clearly formed cusps, ridges/edges, fossae, and pits. Variations of the ideal tooth form can also be viewed. Extracted teeth can also provide the opportunity to view relatively rare dental anomalies as well as more common ones. However, infection control should be of concern with extracted teeth in the student dental professional laboratory setting. Thus persons who collect and inspect extracted teeth should adhere to the infection control procedures as outlined by the Occupational Safety and Health Administration (OSHA) Bloodborne Pathogens Standard as well as considerations presented by more recent research (see Selected References and Additional Resources at the end of these recommendations).

OSHA classifies extracted teeth as clinical specimens because they contain blood with debris, and as such contain potentially infectious material. The biologic material poses a risk of cross-infection (the transfer of pathogenic microorganisms). Hepatitis viruses (HBV and HCV) and the human immunodeficiency virus (HIV) are particularly dangerous. Thus persons who collect, transport, or manipulate extracted teeth should handle them with the same precautions as specimens for biopsy. In addition, extracted teeth may include amalgam restorations, so possible pollutants should be taken into consideration when working with these teeth. Mercury vaporization and exposure is a known health hazard (see later discussion).

If not used for student study or research purposes, extracted teeth should be placed in medical waste containers unless they are returned to the patient and thus are not subject to the OSHA provisions. However, any extracted teeth containing amalgam should not be placed in medical waste containers that use incineration for final disposal as sharps containers routinely do (see later discussion of metal recycling). If keeping the extracted tooth because the dental laboratory wants it for shade or size comparison, the disposal method followed can be the same as that outlined later when used for student study purposes.

Alternatively, extracted teeth kept for research purposes can be soaked in a solution of 10% formalin for two weeks. Tooth immersion in the formalin solution has been found effective in disinfecting both the internal and external structures of the teeth without any structure changes or pollution concerns if amalgam is present, but it will still be necessary to use standard precautions when handling the teeth. However, formalin itself is a hazardous material identified as a potential carcinogen and thus should not be used to routinely disinfect extracted teeth for student study purposes. When using formalin, the manufacturer safety data sheet (SDS) should be reviewed for occupational safety and health concerns and to ensure compliance with OSHA recommendations. Continued research is needed to determine the best method for treating extracted teeth before their use in research.

If kept for student study purposes, OSHA recommends that the "extracted teeth be subject to the containerization and labelling provisions of the bloodborne standard." The associated Centers for Disease Control and Prevention (CDC) guidelines state that extracted teeth should initially be collected in a "securely sealed specimen container" such as a well-constructed, wide-mouthed jar with a secure lid to prevent leakage during transport or storage. For recent basic CDC recommendations, see also extracted-teeth.html.

During the collection, the extracted teeth should be placed in a 10% solution of sodium hypochlorite (bleach diluted 1:10 with tap water) or 3% hydrogen peroxide although recently the CDC states the teeth can be kept moist in a simple solution such as water or saline but need to be cleaned so there is no visible blood or debris (such as with an ultrasonic device), which then can be safely heat-sterilized. Later the contents of the jars can be stored in a 0.2% thymol solution or stay with the water or saline solution if desired per the CDC. At all times, the jars must be clearly marked with a biohazard symbol until sterilization as well as the SDS symbols for sodium hypochlorite and thymol. When using sodium hypochlorite and thymol, the SDS should be reviewed for occupational safety and health concerns.

A recent study to evaluate the efficiency of different sterilization methods on extracted teeth by a systematic review of in vitro randomized controlled trials found that using autoclaving or 10% formalin can still be considered completely efficient and reliable methods for sterilization, while the use alone of 5.25% sodium hypochlorite (bleach), 3% hydrogen peroxide, 2% glutaraldehyde, 0.1% thymol, and boiling to 100°C were considered inefficient and unreliable methods of sterilization for extracted teeth. These chemical agents exert a bactericidal and virucidal action based on oxidation. However, microbiologic tests revealed that not all pathogens are eliminated by them. Past studies also show that ethylene oxide cannot be relied on to sterilize extracted teeth.

It is important to remember that because of the risk of mercury contamination during tooth preparation, extracted teeth with amalgam cannot be saved because they cannot be safely sterilized for viewing for student study. State and local regulations should be consulted regarding the disposal of amalgam; many metal recycling companies will accept extracted teeth with amalgam. Contact a recycler and ask about company policies and about any further handling instructions.

In contrast with formalin preparation for research, this method of using sodium hypochlorite (bleach) or 3% hydrogen peroxide with sterilization for infection control does change the structure of the extracted teeth, but it does not prevent the use of the teeth for general student study purposes. In addition, although extracted teeth can be effectively heat-sterilized, the CDC guidelines state that standard precautions must still be followed at all times (e.g., wearing appropriate personal protective equipment) in handling of these materials by student dental professionals because preclinical educational exercises simulate future clinical experiences.

The disinfection or sterilization method used does affect the fracture resistance of extracted teeth: autoclaved teeth were less resistant to fracture than teeth that were not sterilized or teeth that were chemically disinfected. However, fracture resistance was not reduced enough to lead to tooth fracture during preclinical endodontic procedures. Therefore either processing method may be appropriate for teeth to be used for preclinical endodontic training.

An interesting alternative for formalin seems to be a household vinegar solution. The liquid mainly contains 5% acetic acid in water. The greatest advantage is its accessibility and the ease of use. Teeth immersed in the solution for 1 week were as free of microorganisms as the group stored in 10% formalin and 3% hydrogen peroxide. However, this method requires further investigation in order to establish the proper concentration and its influence on tooth structure. Same is true of the application of an Er:Yag laser or the microwave for disinfecting extracted teeth.

Currently, there is no specific government-sanctioned protocol for the infection control of extracted teeth to be used for student study purposes, except for the recent basic CDC recommendations (see earlier discussion and reference link). However, these effective methods for the infection control of extracted teeth have been determined and found to be acceptable in a student dental professional laboratory setting. More in-depth study needs to be completed of less toxic and easily obtained preparations for controlling infection from extracted teeth for student study purposes instead of having to use sodium hypochlorite, formalin, and thymol.

Method for Extracted Tooth Preparation for Student Study Purposes

Step 1. Use appropriate personal protective equipment as outlined within the standard infection control precautions during preparation of the extracted teeth. Open the collection jars and pour the used sodium hypochlorite (bleach) solution as well as 3% hydrogen peroxide or water or saline solution per the CDC into the local access to the sewer, replacing the older solution with a new 10% sodium hypochlorite (bleach) solution as well as 3% hydrogen peroxide or if desired use water or saline solution per the CDC. The new solution should be left standing, surrounding the collected teeth in the jar, for at least 30 minutes.

Step 2. Using cotton pliers, place collected teeth on several layers of paper towels on a tray to protect work surfaces. Pour the newer sodium hypochlorite (bleach) solution as well as 3% hydrogen peroxide or water or saline solution per the CDC into the local access to the sewer, and discard collection jars and lids in any trash receptacle.

Step 3. Separate the teeth using cotton pliers, and place any teeth to be discarded, such as those with amalgam restorations, into a closed, labeled wide-mouthed jar with new 10% sodium hypochlorite (bleach) solution as well as 3% hydrogen peroxide or stay with water or saline solution if desired per the CDC, and proceed to dispose of properly (see earlier discussion).

Step 4. Place the remaining teeth to be stored into a clear zipper-lock plastic bag with a new 10% sodium hypochlorite (bleach) solution as well as 3% hydrogen peroxide or stay with the water or saline solution if desired per the CDC. Place the closed bag in an ultrasonic machine for 30 minutes to clean the teeth from visble blood and debris. Pour solution from the bag down the local access to the sewer.

Step 5. Teeth should then be covered with a wet paper towel to maintain moisture. Place teeth in plastic autoclave bags, and tape them closed. Heat-sterilize the teeth in an autoclave machine for 40 minutes at the proper temperature and pressure. Discard work materials in the biohazard waste receptacle, and wash hands. Spray tray with germicidal detergent and allow to fully dry.

Step 6. Place the sterilized teeth into clear wide-mouthed jars, so that teeth can be viewed in storage after filling with 0.2% thymol solution before closing with a secure lid or stay with the water or saline solution if desired per the CDC since the teeth are now sterilized. Label jars according to OSHA standards with SDS symbols for thymol if used. Store the teeth under the solution at all times so that they will not dry out and crack.

Step 7. As teeth are needed for examination, they can be removed from the jars with cotton pliers using the appropriate personal protective equipment and rinsed with tap water, soaked in a container of tap water, and rinsed again.

Selected References and Additional Resources

ADA Council on Scientific Affairs: Mercury Hygiene guidelines, *J Am Dent Assoc* 134:1498-1499, 2003.

Attam K, Talwar S, Yadav S, Miglani S: Comparative analysis of the effect of autoclaving and 10% formalin storage on extracted teeth: a microleakage evaluation, *J Conserv Dent* 12:26-30, 2009.

Batchu H, Chou H, Rakowski D, Fan PL: The effect of disinfectants and line cleaners on the release of mercury from amalgam, *J Am Dent Assoc* 137:1419-1425, 2006.

Centers for Disease Control and Prevention: *Guidelines for Infection Control in Dental Health-Care Settings—2003.* MMWR 2003;52(No. RR-17):1–76.

Centers for Disease Control and Prevention: 2003 CDC infection control recommendations for dental health-care settings. *Compend Contin Educ Dent* 25(1 Suppl):43-48, 50-53, 2003.

Centers for Disease Control and Prevention: *Summary of Infection Prevention Practices in Dental Settings: Basic Expectations for Safe Care.* Atlanta, GA: Centers for Disease Control and Prevention, US Dept of Health and Human Services, October 2016.

Chandki R, Mar Ru, Gunwal M, et al: A comparison of different methods for disinfection or sterilization of extracted human teeth to be used for dental education purposes, *World J Dent* 4(1):29-31, 2013.

Dominici JT, Eleazer PD, Clark SJ, Staat RH, Scheetz JP: Disinfection/sterilization of extracted teeth for dental student use, *J Dent Educ* 65:1278-1280, 2001.

Hashemipour MA, Mozafarinia R, Mirzadeh A, et al: Knowledge, attitudes, and performance of dental students in relation to sterilization/disinfection methods of extracted human teeth, *Dent Res J* 10(4): 482-488, 2013.

Hope CK, Griffiths DA, Prior DM. Finding an alternative to formalin for sterilization of extracted teeth for teaching purposes. *J Dent Educ* 77(1):68-71, 2013.

Kumar M, Sequeira PS, Peter S, Bhat GK: Sterilization of extracted human teeth for educational use, *Indian J Med Microbiol* 23(4):256-258, 2005.

Lee JJ, Nettey-Marbell A, Cook A, Pimenta LA, Leonard R, Ritter AV: The effect of storage medium and sterilization on dentin bond strengths, *J Am Dent Assoc* 138:1599-1603, 2007.

Lolayekar NV, Bhat SV, Bhat SS: Disinfection methods of extracted human teeth, *Oral Health Comm Dent* (2):27-29, 2007.

Michaud PL, Maleki M, Mello I: Effect of different disinfection/sterilization methods on risk of fracture of teeth used in preclinical dental education, *J Dent Educ* 82(1):84-87, 2018.

Nawrocka A, Łukomska-Szymańska M. Extracted human teeth and their utility in dental research. Recommendations on proper preservation: A literature review. *Dent Med Probl.* 56(2):185-190, 2019.

Parsell DE, Karns L, Buchanan WT, Johnson RB: Mercury release during autoclave sterilization of amalgam, *J Dent Educ* 60(5):453-458, 1996.

Salem-Milani A, Zand V, Asghari-Jafarabadi M, et al: The effect of protocol for disinfection of extracted teeth recommended by Center for Disease Control (CDC) on microhardness of enamel and dentin, *J Clin Exp Dent* 7(5):e552-e556, 2015.

Tijare MJ, et al: Vinegar as a disinfectant of extracted human teeth for dental educational use, *Oral Maxillofac Pathol* 18(1):14-18, 2014.

U.S. Department of Labor, Occupational Safety and Health Administration: 29 CFR Part 1910.1030. Occupational exposure to bloodborne pathogens; needlestick and other sharps injuries; final rule, *Federal Register*

66:5317-5325, 2001. Updated from and including 29 CFR Part 1910.1030. Occupational exposure to blood-borne pathogens; final rule, *Federal Register* 56:64003-64182, 1991.

U.S. Department of Labor, Occupational Safety and Health Administration: Enforcement procedures for the occupational exposure to bloodborne pathogens. Washington, DC: U.S. Department of Labor, Occupational Safety and Health Administration. Directive No. CPL 02–02–069, 2001.

U.S. Environmental Protection Agency. Data from the 2011 National Emissions Inventory, Version 1, 2014.

Western SJ, Dicksit DD: A systematic review of randomized controlled trials on sterilization methods of extracted human teeth, *J Conserv Dent* 19(4):343-346, 2016.

UNIT I: OROFACIAL STRUCTURES

Note: Answers can be obtained from your instructor and their Evolve Resources

Matching

Match each item below with its best short description; each single item can only be matched once.

a.	Lymph nodes	k.	Body	u.	Buccal fat pad
b.	Exostoses	l.	Parathyroid glands	v.	Alae
c.	Periodontal ligament	m.	Vermilion zone	w.	Maxillary sinus
d.	Vestibules	n.	Mandibular symphysis	x.	Temporomandibular joint
e.	Labial frenum	o.	Fordyce spots	y.	Maxillary tuberosity
f.	Enamel	p.	Mandibular notch	z.	Linea alba
g.	External nose	q.	Anterior teeth		
h.	Parotid papilla	r.	Vertical dimension		
i.	Philtrum	s.	Buccal		
j.	Rami	t.	Tori		

1. Need to be recorded in patient's chart if palpable _____

2. Main feature of nasal region on face _____

3. Terminates in thicker area of midline of upper lip at tubercle _____

4. Mandibular bony feature between coronoid process and condyle _____

5. Division of face into thirds from forehead to chin _____

6. Glands that can be palpated close to or within thyroid gland _____

7. Marking midline of mandible of lower face _____

8. Plural of ramus that is present as mandibular bony feature _____

9. Upper and lower horseshoe-shaped spaces in oral cavity _____

10. Loss of this lip surface feature with excessive solar damage _____

11. Structure orientation that is closest to inner cheek _____

12. Oral feature at midline between labial mucosa and alveolar mucosa on both dental arches _____

13. Elevation of tissue on inner part of buccal mucosa opposite permanent maxillary second molar _____

14. Small yellow elevations within oral mucosa that increase with age _____

15. Heavy horizontal part of maxilla or mandible inferior to roots of teeth _____

16. Attaches tooth to bony surface of alveoli _____

17. Hard outer layer of crown of tooth _____

18. Incisors and canines as group within both dentitions _____

19. Slow-growing masses in premolar area noted on radiographs _____

20. Maxillary arch bony growths that may be related to occlusal trauma _____

21. Acts as protective cushion during mastication _____

22. White ridge of hyperkeratinization extending horizontally where teeth occlude _____

23. Tissue-covered bony elevation just distal to last tooth of maxillary arch _____

24. Nares bounded laterally by winglike cartilaginous structures _____

25. Structure inferior to zygomatic arch and just anterior to external ear _____

26. Structure contained within body of maxilla _____

True or False

Assign the statement below as either true or false.

1. To palpate the lower jaw moving at the temporomandibular joint on a patient, a finger is placed on top of the temporal bone on each side during movement. _____

2. On the midline of the upper lip extending downward from the nasal septum is a vertical groove, the philtrum. _____

3. The bone underlying the mental region is the mandible, or lower jaw. _____

4. At the sides of the neck is the hyoid bone, which is suspended in the neck. _____

5. Inferior to the hyoid bone is the thyroid cartilage, which is the prominence of the larynx. _____

6. The thyroid gland, an endocrine gland, can be palpated on a patient within the midline cervical area. _____

7. The upper and lower lips meet at each corner of the mouth at the labial commissure. _____

8. The bony support for the cheek is the temporomandibular joint. _____

9. The nares are separated by the midline nasal septum. _____

10. The eyeball and all its supporting structures are contained in the orbit of the skull. _____

11. The zygomatic arch extends from just below the lateral margin of the eye toward the middle part of the external nose. _____

12. Those lingual structures closest to the palate are palatal. _____

13. Deep within each vestibule is the vestibular fornix, where the pinkish labial mucosa or buccal mucosa meets the redder alveolar mucosa. _____

14. An excess amount of linea alba on either the buccal mucosa or tongue can be associated with certain oral parafunctional habits. _____

15. The maxilla is a single bone with a movable articulation with the temporal bones at each temporomandibular joint. _____

16. The vertically placed canine eminence is especially prominent on each side of the maxilla. _____

17. The dense pad of tissue located just distal to the last tooth of the mandibular arch is the retromolar pad. _____

18. The permanent maxillary anterior teeth are supplied by the anterior superior alveolar artery; the permanent maxillary posterior teeth are supplied by the posterior superior alveolar artery. _____

19. The permanent mandibular teeth are supplied by branches of the anterior superior alveolar artery. _____

20. The alveolar process is the bony extension for both the maxilla and mandible that contain each alveolus. _____

21. The inner parts of the lips are lined by a pinkish buccal mucosa. _____

22. Both the labial and buccal mucosa may vary in coloration, as do other regions of the oral mucosa, in individuals with pigmented skin. _____

23. The interdental gingiva is the gingival tissue between adjacent teeth adjoining attached gingiva. _____

24. The inner surface of the gingival tissue where each tooth faces a space is the gingival sulcus. _____

25. The inside of the mouth is also known as the *oral cavity proper*. _____

26. Posteriorly, the opening from the oral cavity proper into the pharynx is the palate. _____

27. The palatine tonsils are located on the lateral side of the tongue. _____

28. A midline ridge of tissue on the hard palate is the retromolar pad. _____

29. The palatine rugae are firm irregular ridges of tissue radiating from the incisive papilla and median palatine raphe. _____

30. The sulcus terminalis separates the base from the body of the tongue. _____

31. If disruption of the vermilion zone and its mucocutaneous junction at the vermilion border has been caused by a traumatic incident, noting it in the patient record is important given that the rest of the oral cavity may be affected. _____

32. If considering the diagnosis of cancer, this can be verified only with tissue biopsy and microscopic examination. _____

33. The risk of cancerous changes with the lips can be increased only with chronic alcohol use and not with chronic tobacco use. _____

34. The protection of only the lower lip with sunscreen is important because sun exposure increases the risk of cancerous changes. _____

35. Visible surface changes may be caused by underlying associated histologic tissue changes. _____

36. The face can be divided vertically into fourths, and this perspective is considered the vertical dimension of the face. _____

37. A discussion of vertical dimension allows a comparison of the divisions of the face for functional and esthetic purposes using the guidelines of the Golden Proportions. _____

38. Surface changes in the features of the face and neck may be caused by underlying developmental disturbances. _____

39. Knowledge of the surface features of the face and neck additionally helps dental professionals understand the associated developmental pattern. _____

40. The variations among individuals are only what should be noted and not the changes in a particular individual. _____

41. To visualize the area of focus successfully for the dental professional, it is important to know the boundaries, terminology, and divisions of the oral cavity as well as the pharynx. _____

42. Some degree of variation can be possible in the oral cavity and visible divisions of the pharynx. _____

43. A change in any tissue or associated structure in a patient may signal a condition of clinical significance and must be noted in the patient record as well as correctly followed up by the examining dental professional. _____

44. Exostoses appear on radiographs as radiopaque (light) areas. _____

45. A variation present usually on the facial surface of the alveolar process of the maxillary arch is considered a palatal torus. _____

46. Mandibular tori are usually present bilaterally in the area of the premolars and can appear as lobulated or nodular raised areas. _____

47. More serious pathology of the palate, such as a history of cleft palate, needs to be noted in the patient record because of its impact on dental care. _____

48. The laryngopharynx is visible in most cases to the dental professional. _____

49. The pharynx has two divisions, the oropharynx and the laryngopharynx. _____

50. The structure of the fauces marks the boundary between the oropharynx and the oral cavity proper. _____

Ordering

Place the following items in the correct order as indicated.

1. In what order should these facial surface features be placed, going from superior to inferior on the face?
   _____ a. Infraorbital region
   _____ b. Mental region
   _____ c. Orbital region
   _____ d. Frontal region

2. In what order should these oral region features be placed, going from the outer part to inner part of the upper lip?
   _____ a. Vermilion zone
   _____ b. Mucocutaneous junction
   _____ c. Tubercle of the upper lip
   _____ d. Philtrum

3. In what order should these facial surface features be placed, going from medial to lateral on the face?
   _____ a. Nasal region
   _____ b. External ear
   _____ c. Infraorbital region
   _____ d. Zygomatic region

4. In what order should these facial surface features be placed, going from superior to inferior on the face?
   _____ a. Philtrum
   _____ b. Root of the nose
   _____ c. Nares
   _____ d. Apex of the nose

5. In what order should these neck surface features be placed, going from superior to inferior on the neck?
   _____ a. Thyroid cartilage
   _____ b. Hyoid bone
   _____ c. Mandible
   _____ d. Thyroid gland

6. In what order should these facial surface features be placed, going from medial to lateral on the face?
   _____ a. Mandibular condyle
   _____ b. Labial commissures
   _____ c. Mandibular notch
   _____ d. Coronoid process

7. In what order should these oral cavity features be placed, going from superior to inferior on the maxillary arch?

    _____ a. Attached gingiva

    _____ b. Marginal gingiva

    _____ c. Mucogingival junction

    _____ d. Alveolar mucosa

8. In what order should these oral cavity features be placed, going from anterior to posterior on the palate?

    _____ a. Palatal rugae

    _____ b. Incisive papilla

    _____ c. Maxillary incisors

    _____ d. Attached gingiva

9. In what order should these oral cavity features be placed, going from anterior to posterior on the dorsal surface of the tongue?

    _____ a. Body of the tongue

    _____ b. Apex of the tongue

    _____ c. Base of the tongue

    _____ d. Sulcus terminalis

10. In what order should these features of both the larynx and pharynx be placed, going from superior to inferior within the neck area?

    _____ a. Nasopharynx

    _____ b. Larynx

    _____ c. Oropharynx

    _____ d. Laryngopharynx

UNIT II: DENTAL EMBRYOLOGY

Matching

Match each item with the best short description below; each single item can only be matched once.

a.	Cloacal membrane	k.	Mesoderm	u.	Meckel cartilage
b.	Differentiation	l.	Morphogenesis	v.	Secondary palate
c.	Ectoderm	m.	Neural crest cells	w.	Cap stage
d.	Embryonic period	n.	Neuroectoderm	x.	Primary palate
e.	Endoderm	o.	Oropharyngeal membrane	y.	Supernumerary teeth
f.	Fetal period	p.	Placenta	z.	Frontonasal process
g.	Fusion	q.	Preimplantation period		
h.	Induction	r.	Primitive streak		
i.	Maturation	s.	Proliferation		
j.	Mesenchyme	t.	Somites		

1. Period when fertilization and implantation occur _____

2. Period involving embryo growing into fetus _____

3. Second week to eighth week of prenatal development _____

4. Action of one group of cells on another that leads to establishment of developmental pathway in responding tissue _____

5. Controlled cellular growth and accumulation of by-products _____

6. Change in identical embryonic cells to become distinct, noted both structurally and functionally _____

7. Development of specific tissue structure or differing form due to embryonic cell migration and inductive interactions _____

8. Attainment of adult function and size due to proliferation, differentiation, and morphogenesis _____

9. Originates directly from epiblast layer _____

10. Future dermis, muscle, bone _____

11. Layer of cuboidal cells within embryo _____

12. Considered by many histologists to be fourth embryonic layer _____

13. Prenatal organ that joins pregnant woman and developing embryo _____

14. Furrowed rod-shaped thickening in middle of embryonic disc _____

15. Differentiates to form most of connective tissue of head _____

16. Location of future primitive mouth of embryo _____

17. Location of future terminal end of embryo's digestive tract _____

18. Specialized group of cells that differentiates from ectoderm _____

19. Elimination of groove between two adjacent swellings of tissue or processes on embryo surface _____

20. Mesoderm that additionally differentiates and begins to divide into paired cuboidal aggregates of cells _____

21. Most disappears as bony mandible forms by intramembranous ossification _____

22. Forms as bulge of tissue at most cephalic end of embryo _____

23. Initially serves as partial separation between developing oral cavity proper and nasal cavity _____

24. Will give rise to posterior two-thirds of hard palate _____

25. Abnormal initiation may result in development of one or more extra teeth _____

26. Stage of unequal growth in different parts of tooth bud _____

True or False

Assign the statement below as either true or false.

1. The face and its related tissue begin to form during the sixth week of prenatal development. _____

2. All three embryonic layers are involved in facial development. _____

3. Facial development is completed for the most part during the twelfth week of prenatal development. _____

4. The overall growth of the face is in a superior and posterior direction in relationship to the cranial base. _____

5. The stomodeum initially appears as a shallow depression in the embryonic surface ectoderm at the cephalic end. _____

6. Oral epithelium is derived from ectoderm as a result of embryonic folding. _____

7. The paired maxillary processes fuse at the midline to form the mandibular arch. _____

8. The placodes are rounded areas of specialized, thickened ectoderm found at the location of developing special sense organs. _____

9. The paired medial nasal processes also fuse internally and grow inferiorly on the inside of the stomodeum, forming the intermaxillary segment. _____

10. The upper lip is formed when each maxillary process fuses with each nearby medial nasal process. _____

11. The beginnings of the embryo's hollow tube are derived from the anterior part of the midgut. _____

12. The stacked bilateral outer swellings of tissue that appear inferior to the stomodeum and include the mandibular arch are the branchial or pharyngeal pouches. _____

13. Palatal fusion allows the fusion of swellings or tissue from different surfaces of the embryo. _____

14. The intermaxillary segment gives rise to the secondary palate. _____

15. The secondary palate will give rise to the anterior one-third of the hard palate. _____

16. In the future, the neural crest cells will become involved in the formation of components of the nervous system, melanocyte pigment cells. _____

17. The tongue develops during the fourth to eighth weeks of prenatal development. _____

18. Tongue development begins as a triangular median swelling, the tuberculum impar. _____

19. The copula is formed from the fusion of mesenchyme of mainly the third and parts of the fourth branchial or pharyngeal arches. _____

20. The foramen cecum is the beginning of the thymus. _____

21. The oral epithelium grows deeper into the ectomesenchyme and is induced to produce a layer called the dental membrane. _____

22. A depression results in the deepest part of each tooth bud of dental lamina and forms the enamel knot. _____

23. The dental papilla will produce the future dentin and pulp for the inner part of the tooth. _____

24. Three embryologic structures, the enamel organ, dental papilla, and dental sac, are considered together to be the tooth germ. _____

25. After the inner enamel epithelium differentiates into preameloblasts, the outer cells of the dental papilla are induced by the preameloblasts to differentiate into ameloblasts. _____

26. Developmental disturbances can occur within each stage of odontogenesis, affecting the physiologic processes taking place. _____

27. The initial teeth for both dentitions develop in the anterior maxillary region. _____

28. The primary dentition develops during only the embryonic period of prenatal development. _____

29. The second stage of odontogenesis is considered bud stage and occurs at the beginning of the eighth week of prenatal development for the primary dentition. _____

30. The dental sac will produce the periodontium, the supporting tissue types of the tooth. _____

31. Dental professionals need to have a clear understanding of the major events of prenatal development in order to understand the development of the structures of the face, neck, and oral cavity and the underlying relationships among these structures. _____

32. Prenatal development begins with the start of pregnancy and continues until the formation of the embryo. _____

33. Developmental disturbances that involve the orofacial structures as well as other parts of the body can include congenital malformations. _____

34. Noninvasive prenatal testing is a cell-free fetal DNA testing that involves a simple blood draw from the pregnant woman. _____

35. Environmental agents and factors involved in causing congenital malformations can include infections and radiation but not drugs. _____

36. Women of reproductive age should avoid teratogens to protect the developing infant from possible congenital malformations. _____

37. Down syndrome is where an extra chromosome number 12 is present after meiotic division. _____

38. Implantation of the zygote may also occur outside the uterus with an ectopic pregnancy. _____

39. Ectodermal dysplasia has a hereditary etiology and presents with abnormalities of the teeth, skin, hair, nails, eyes, facial structure, and glands. _____

40. If there is failure of migration of the neural crest cells to the neck region, Treacher Collins syndrome develops in the fetus. _____

41. Systemic tetracycline antibiotic therapy of the pregnant woman can act as a teratogenic drug during the fetal period. _____

42. A cleft lip results from a failure of the endoderm to grow beneath the mesoderm to obliterate any grooves between these processes or even a deficiency or absence of mesenchyme in the area. _____

43. The growth and development of the thymus is complete at birth. _____

44. Most congenital malformations in the neck originate during transformation of the branchial or pharyngeal apparatus into its mature derivatives. _____

45. The first branchial or pharyngeal grooves occasionally do not become obliterated and thus parts remain to form a branchial cleft cyst. _____

46. Failure of fusion of the palatal shelves with the primary palate, with each other, or both results in cleft palate. _____

47. Abnormally large teeth result in microdontia; abnormally small teeth result in macrodontia.

_____

48. Misplaced ameloblasts can migrate to the surface of the root to produce an enamel pearl. _____

49. Developmental root anatomy variants may involve linguogingival or palatogingival grooves as well as proximal root grooves. _____

50. A primary tooth often starts to erupt before the permanent tooth is fully shed, which may create complications in spacing. _____

Ordering

Place the following items in the correct order as indicated.

1. In what order should these events during prenatal development be noted, going from earlier to later in time span?

    _____ a. Conception

    _____ b. Preimplantation period

    _____ c. Fetal period

    _____ d. Embryonic period

2. In what order should these events occurring during prenatal development be noted, going from earlier to later in time span?

    _____ a. Mitosis

    _____ b. Implantation

    _____ c. Meiosis

    _____ d. Sperm and egg union

3. In what order should these structures present during prenatal development be noted, going from earlier to later in time span?

    _____ a. Fetus

    _____ b. Embryo

    _____ c. Blastocyst

    _____ d. Zygote

4. In what order should these prenatal structures be placed, going from closest to farthest in relationship to the endometrium lining the uterus?

    _____ a. Amniotic cavity

    _____ b. Hypoblast layer

    _____ c. Epiblast layer

    _____ d. Yolk sac

5. In what order should these prenatal structures be placed, going from superior to inferior in relationship to the embryo?

    _____ a. Midgut

    _____ b. Hindgut

    _____ c. Foregut

    _____ d. Oropharyngeal membrane

6. In what order should these structures present during prenatal development be noted, going from earlier to later in time span?

    _____ a. Stomodeum

    _____ b. Mandibular processes

    _____ c. Mandibular arch

    _____ d. Primitive mouth

7. In what order should these prenatal structures be placed, going from superior to inferior in relationship to the embryo?

   _____ a. Hyoid arch

   _____ b. Third branchial or pharyngeal arch

   _____ c. Mandibular arch

   _____ d. Fourth branchial or pharyngeal arch

8. In what order should these prenatal structures be placed, going from superior to inferior in relationship to the embryo?

   _____ a. Frontonasal process

   _____ b. Maxillary processes

   _____ c. Mandibular arch

   _____ d. Stomodeum

9. In what order should these structures present during palatal development be noted, going from earlier to later in time span?

   _____ a. Primary palate

   _____ b. Intermaxillary segment

   _____ c. Palatal shelves

   _____ d. Secondary palate

10. In what order should these structures present during tongue development be noted, going from earlier to later in time span?

    _____ a. Copula

    _____ b. Lateral lingual swellings

    _____ c. Epiglottic swelling

    _____ d. Tuberculum impar

11. In what order should these events during odontogenesis be noted, going from earlier to later in time span?

    _____ a. Bud stage

    _____ b. Cap stage

    _____ c. Initiation stage

    _____ d. Bell stage

12. In what order should these layers of the enamel organ be placed, going from the outer part to inner part in relationship to the overall tooth?

    _____ a. Outer enamel epithelium

    _____ b. Stellate reticulum

    _____ c. Inner enamel epithelium

    _____ d. Stratum intermedium

UNIT III: DENTAL HISTOLOGY

Matching

Match each item below with its best short description; each single item can only be matched once.

a.	Anaphase	k.	Mucoperiosteum	u.	Interglobular dentin
b.	Basement membrane	l.	Nucleoplasm	v.	Lamina dura
c.	Cell	m.	Organ	w.	Sulcular epithelium
d.	Connective tissue	n.	Organelles	x.	Fibroblast
e.	Cytoplasm	o.	Prophase	y.	Gingival recession
f.	Epithelium	p.	Rete ridges	z.	Attrition
g.	Granulation tissue	q.	System		
h.	Histology	r.	Telophase		
i.	Interphase	s.	Tissue		
j.	Metaphase	t.	Von Ebner		

1. Study of microscopic structure and function of cells and tissue _____

2. Smallest living unit of organization _____

3. Collection of similarly specialized cells _____

4. Independent body part formed from tissue _____

5. Organs functioning together _____

6. Semifluid part contained within cell membrane boundary _____

7. Chromatin condenses into chromosomes _____

8. Mitotic spindle forms during cell division _____

9. Migration of chromatids to opposite poles by mitotic spindle _____

10. Reappearance of nuclear membrane _____

11. Cells between divisions involved in this time period _____

12. Specialized metabolically active structures within cell _____

13. Fluid part within nucleus of cell _____

14. Tissue type that covers and lines external and internal body surfaces _____

15. Extensions of epithelium into connective tissue _____

16. Thin acellular chemical-based structure located between any form of epithelium and its underlying connective tissue _____

17. Most abundant type of basic tissue by weight _____

18. Immature connective tissue with few fibers and increased amount of blood vessels _____

19. Consisting of mucous membrane combined with periosteum of adjacent bone _____

20. Glands present in submucosa deep to lamina propria of circumvallate lingual papillae _____

21. Wearing of hard tissue as result of tooth-to-tooth contact _____

22. Can cause root dentin to be exposed with thin layer of cementum lost _____

23. Only primary mineralization has occurred within predentin _____

24. Part of alveolar bone proper present on radiographs _____

25. Most common cell in periodontal ligament _____

26. Stands away from tooth creating gingival sulcus _____

True or False

Assign the statement below as either true or false.

1. The interdental gingiva assumes a nonvisible concave form between the facial and lingual gingival surfaces called the col. _____

2. Healthy attached gingiva is pinkish in color, with some areas of melanin pigmentation possible. _____

3. In some cases, a free gingival groove separates the sulcular gingiva from the marginal gingiva. _____

4. The dentogingival junction is the direct junction between the tooth surface and the periodontal ligament. _____

5. The sulcular epithelium is of an orthokeratinized type, with its cells tightly packed. _____

6. Before the eruption of the tooth and after enamel maturation, the ameloblasts secrete a basal lamina on the surface that serves as a part of the primary epithelial attachment. _____

7. An endocrine gland is a gland having a duct associated with it. _____

8. Saliva also supplies the minerals for subgingival calculus formation. _____

9. Mucoserous acini have both a group of mucous cells surrounding the lumen and a serous demilune. _____

10. More than one myoepithelial cell can sometimes be found on a single acinus. _____

11. The submandibular salivary gland is the smallest, most diffuse, and only unencapsulated major salivary gland. _____

12. The parathyroid glands are visible or palpable during an extraoral examination of a patient. _____

13. Tissue fluid drains from the surrounding region into the lymphatic vessels as lymph. _____

14. Each lymphatic nodule has a germinal center containing many immature lymphocytes. _____

15. Intraoral tonsillar tissue consists of nonencapsulated masses of lymphoid tissue located in the lamina propria of the oral mucosa. _____

16. The palatine tonsils are four rounded masses of variable size located between the anterior and posterior faucial pillars. _____

17. The lingual tonsil is an indistinct layer of diffuse lymphoid tissue located on the lateral surface of the tongue. _____

18. Each lateral wall of the nasal cavity has three projecting structures or nasal conchae that extend inward. _____

19. The nasal cavity is lined by a respiratory mucosa, like the rest of the respiratory system. _____

20. The moist mucus forms a deep invasive system in the respiratory mucosa. _____

21. The underlying histologic states of its components provide a clue to the clinical features noted visibly with the periodontium, whether in a healthy or diseased state. _____

22. The mature cementum consists of mainly calcium hydroxyapatite with the chemical formula of $Ca_{10}(PO_4)_6(OH)_2$. _____

23. The trabecular bone appears less uniformly radiopaque and more porous than the uniformly radiopaque lamina dura. _____

24. With the loss of teeth, a patient becomes edentulous, either partially or completely. _____

25. During the chronic advanced type of periodontal disease of periodontitis, the basal bone is always lost. _____

26. The epithelial rests of Malassez are present within the alveolar process but can become cystic. _____

27. The periodontal ligament is wider near the apex and cervix of the tooth. _____

28. During mastication and speech, certain forces are exerted on a tooth, such as rotational, tilting, extrusive, or intrusive. _____

29. The interradicular group of the alveolodental ligament is found only between the alveolar crests of neighboring teeth. _____

30. The dentogingival ligament is the most extensive of the gingival fiber group. _____

31. A type of intercellular junction is formed by a desmosome, which involves an attachment of a cell to an adjacent noncellular surface. _____

32. The turnover time is faster for all types of connective tissue as compared to epithelium. _____

33. The details of the basement membrane are not seen when it is viewed by scanning or lower-power magnification. _____

34. The amount of scar tissue varies, depending on the type and size of the injury, amount of granulation tissue, and movement of tissue after injury. _____

35. By age 10, the skin begins to deteriorate and by the age of 20 is in a rapid state of degradation because of the aging process. _____

36. Microscopically a cross-section of bone demonstrates layers related to its development that look like growth rings in a tree. _____

37. Changes such as hyperkeratinization are reversible if the source of the injury is removed, but it takes time for the keratin to be shed by the tissue. _____

38. The two types of taste bud cells are the supporting cells and the taste cells. _____

39. The lesion of geographic tongue shows the sensitivity of the fungiform lingual papillae to changes in their environment. _____

40. The pigmentation of both the oral mucosa and skin may increase with certain endocrine diseases. _____

41. All regions of the oral cavity have a faster turnover time than the skin. _____

42. The formation of more scar tissue in the oral mucosa is useful both esthetically and functionally when oral or periodontal surgery is performed. _____

43. The biologic width describes the combined heights of the suprabony soft tissue, which is attached to the part of the tooth coronal to the crest of the alveolar bone. _____

44. The gingival biotype is the thickness of the gingiva within the mesiodistal dimension. _____

45. The junctional epithelium is attached on the other side to the laminal propria of nearby gingiva, as is the sulcular epithelium. _____

46. The junctional epithelium has only one basal lamina and it faces the tooth. _____

47. The amount of gingival overgrowth through drug-influenced gingival hyperplasia is related to the drug dosage. _____

48. The decreased production of saliva is considered xerostomia and can result in dry mouth or hyposalivation. _____

49. A common developmental disturbance is the deepened pit and groove patterns on the facial surface of anterior teeth and on the root surface of posterior teeth. _____

50. An unwanted side effect of rapid orthodontic therapy can be root apex resorption, reducing the overall length of the tooth. _____

Ordering

Place the following items in the correct order as indicated.

1. In what order should these cellular structures be placed, going from outer part to inner part of the cell?

   _____ a. Cell membrane

   _____ b. Nucleolus

   _____ c. Nucleus

   _____ d. Nuclear membrane

2. In what order should these components of the body be noted, going from a simple to a more complex type of organization?

   _____ a. Cell

   _____ b. Organ

   _____ c. Tissue

   _____ d. System

3. In what order should these phases present during mitosis be noted, going from earlier to later in time span?

   _____ a. Anaphase

   _____ b. Prophase

   _____ c. Metaphase

   _____ d. Telophase

4. In what order should these bone layers be placed, going from superficial to deeper layers in the tissue?

   _____ a. Compact bone

   _____ b. Endosteum

   _____ c. Periosteum

   _____ d. Cancellous bone

5. In what order should these steps present during endochondrial ossification be noted, going from earlier to later in time span?

   _____ a. Formation of primary ossification centers

   _____ b. Osteoblasts penetrate cartilage

   _____ c. Production of osteoid in layers

   _____ d. Cartilage disintegrates

6. In what order should these components of skeletal muscle be placed, going from superficial to deeper layers in relationship to the muscle bundle?

   _____ a. Myofilaments

   _____ b. Myofibers

   _____ c. Myofibrils

   _____ d. Muscle fascicles

7. In what order should these layers of orthokeratinized stratified squamous epithelium be placed, going from superficial to deeper layers in the tissue?

   _____ a. Keratin layer

   _____ b. Basal layer

   _____ c. Prickle layer

   _____ d. Granular layer

8. In what order should these salivary glands be noted, going from largest to smallest as related to individual size?

   _____ a. von Ebner gland

   _____ b. Submandibular gland

   _____ c. Parotid gland

   _____ d. Sublingual gland

9. In what order should these components of salivary glands be placed, going from larger to smaller in size as well as superficial to deeper within the gland?

_____ a. Lobes

_____ b. Acini

_____ c. Capsule

_____ d. Lobules

10. In what order should these components of salivary glands be placed, going from superficial near the capsule to deeper in the gland?

_____ a. Intercalated duct

_____ b. Acinus

_____ c. Striated duct

_____ d. Excretory duct

11. In what order should these components of the thyroid gland be placed, going from larger to smaller in size as well as superficial to deeper within the gland?

_____ a. Lobes

_____ b. Follicles

_____ c. Capsule

_____ d. Lobules

12. In what order should these components of a lymph node be noted, going the same way as the flow of lymph entering and exiting the node?

_____ a. Efferent vessel

_____ b. Lymphatic vessel

_____ c. Afferent vessel

_____ d. Hilus

13. In what order should these components of a lymph node be placed, going from larger to smaller in size as well as superficial to deeper within the node?

_____ a. Lymphatic nodule

_____ b. Trabeculae

_____ c. Capsule

_____ d. Germinal center

14. In what order should these events involving the ameloblasts during odontogenesis be placed, going from earlier to later in time span?

_____ a. Forming enamel matrix from Tomes process

_____ b. Actively transporting materials for mineralization

_____ c. Becoming part of reduced enamel epithelium

_____ d. Removing water and organic material from enamel

15. In what order should these zones in pulp be placed, going from the outer pulpal wall near the dentin to the inner part of the pulp?

_____ a. Pulpal core

_____ b. Cell-rich zone

_____ c. Cell-free zone

_____ d. Odontoblastic layer

16. In what order should these fiber groups of the alveolodental ligament of the periodontal ligament be placed, going from the cementoenamel junction to the tooth apex?

_____ a. Horizontal group

_____ b. Oblique group

_____ c. Alveolar crest group

_____ d. Apical group

UNIT IV: DENTAL ANATOMY

Matching

Match each item below with its best short description; each single item can only be matched once.

a.	Anatomic root	k.	Furcation	u.	Occlusal table
b.	Bicuspid	l.	Mamelons	v.	Transverse ridge
c.	Bifurcated	m.	Occlusion	w.	Trifurcated
d.	Bruxism	n.	Overjet	x.	Curve of Wilson
e.	Centric relationship	o.	Palmer Notation Method	y.	Wisdom
f.	Cervical ridge	p.	Primate spaces	z.	Articular fossa
g.	Cingulum	q.	Sextant		
h.	Contact	r.	Adult teeth		
i.	Cuspids	s.	Supplemental grooves		
j.	Diastema	t.	Supporting cusps		

1. Other name for permanent dentition that is more commonly used _____

2. Tooth numbering system commonly used during orthodontic therapy _____

3. Used to describe anatomic alignment of teeth and relationship to rest of masticatory system _____

4. Division of each dental arch into three parts based on relationship to midline _____

5. Part of root covered by layer of cementum _____

6. Raised rounded area on cervical third of lingual surface of anterior teeth _____

7. Rounded enamel extensions on incisal ridge from either labial or lingual views _____

8. Mainly viewed as open contact between permanent maxillary central incisors _____

9. Older term for canines that is still commonly used _____

10. Occlusal surface is bordered by marginal ridges to create inner surface _____

11. Joining of two triangular ridges crossing occlusal surface from labial to lingual outline _____

12. Secondary grooves on occlusal surface that appear as shallow and more irregular linear depressions _____

13. Older term for premolar that is still commonly used _____

14. Maxillary first premolars having two root branches _____

15. Common name for third molars _____

16. Area between two or more of the root branches before division from root trunk _____

17. Maxillary molars with three root branches _____

18. Spaces between primary maxillary lateral incisor and canine and between primary mandibular canine and first molar _____

19. Ridge more prominent on primary molars than any similar structure on permanent molar _____

20. Cause of extensive wear of incisal edge of primary incisor _____

21. End point of closure of mandible _____

22. Maxillary dental arch naturally overhanging mandibular arch facially _____

23. Area on proximal surfaces of teeth with same-arch neighbors _____

24. Concave curve that results when frontal section is taken through each set of both maxillary and mandibular molars _____

25. Cusps that function during centric occlusion _____

26. Depression on inferior aspect of temporal bone _____

True or False

Assign the statement below as either true or false.

1. The anteroposterior curvature is called the curve of Wilson, which is produced by the curved alignment of all the teeth and is especially evident when viewing the posterior teeth from the buccal. _____

2. Phase three of arch development begins when the canines wedge themselves between the lateral incisors and the first premolars. _____

3. Open contacts allow for areas of food impaction from opposing cusps, which are called plunging cusps, resulting in trauma to the interdental gingiva. _____

4. Overbite is measured in millimeters with the tip of a periodontal probe. _____

5. If a tooth is lost for a longer period, the neighboring teeth usually become more upright in an effort to fill the edentulous space. _____

6. Triangular grooves separate a marginal ridge from the triangular ridge of a cusp and at their terminations form the triangular fossae. _____

7. The contact area of each of the posterior teeth is wider than anterior teeth, is usually located to the lingual of center, and is nearer the same level on each proximal surface. _____

8. Some inclined planes are functional and thus involved in the occlusion of the teeth. _____

9. The crown of each posterior tooth has an occlusal surface as its masticatory surface, bordered by the raised marginal ridges, which are located on both the facial surface and lingual surface. _____

10. Most permanent maxillary first premolars are trifurcated, having two root branches in the apical third, with a buccal root and a lingual root. _____

11. Permanent maxillary second premolars erupt between 10 and 12 years of age. _____

12. There is one form of permanent mandibular second premolars, the tricuspidate form, which is a three-cusp type. _____

13. The permanent dentition is also sometimes considered the nonsuccedaneous dentition, because all of these permanent teeth succeed primary predecessors. _____

14. The molars, because of their tapered shape and their prominent cusp, function to pierce or tear food during mastication. _____

15. A tooth numbering system that is commonly used in orthodontic therapy is the Palmer Notation Method. _____

16. The joint capsule outer layer is a synovial membrane, which consists of a thin connective tissue with nerves and blood vessels. _____

17. The central area of the temporomandibular joint disc is vascularized and has innervation. _____

18. Lateral deviation of the mandible, or lateral excursion, which involves shifting the lower jaw to one side, occurs during mastication. _____

19. Not all patients with temporomandibular disorders have abnormalities in the joint disc or even in the joint itself; most symptoms seem to originate from the muscles. _____

20. The Palmer Notation Method is also known as the *Military Tooth Numbering System.* _____

21. The permanent dentition period begins with the eruption of the primary mandibular central incisors. _____

22. The mixed dentition period occurs between approximately 6 and 12 years of age. _____

23. A growth center is located in the head of each mandibular condyle before an individual can reach maturity. _____

24. Lateral deviation involves only gliding movements of contralateral temporomandibular joints in their respective joint cavities. _____

25. When the teeth of the occlusion are in the position of centric occlusion, each tooth of one arch is in occlusion with two others in the opposing arch, except for a few teeth. _____

26. Premature contacts are where one or two teeth contact after the other teeth. _____

27. The permanent canine should usually be the only tooth in function during lateral occlusion. _____

28. The permanent central incisors are closest to the midline, and the permanent lateral incisors are the second teeth from the midline. _____

29. The pulp chamber of the permanent maxillary central incisor has two sharp elongations: the mesial and distal pulp horns. _____

30. The lingual surface of the crown of a permanent maxillary lateral incisor is narrower than the labial surface. _____

31. The crown of a permanent mandibular central incisor is quite asymmetrical from the labial view. _____

32. Because of their tapered shape and prominent cusp, the permanent canines function to pierce or tear food during mastication. _____

33. The mesial half of the crown of a permanent maxillary canine resembles a part of a premolar, and the distal half resembles a part of a permanent incisor. _____

34. Like anterior teeth, multirooted permanent premolars and molars originate as a single root on the base of the crown. _____

35. Because the permanent maxillary first molar has a buccal and lingual root, it also has two furcations. _____

36. The lingual cusp is slightly displaced to the distal, which helps distinguish the permanent maxillary right second premolar from the left. _____

37. Both types of permanent mandibular premolars can present difficulties during instrumentation due to narrow lingual surfaces combined with the lingual inclination of the crown. _____

38. The permanent mandibular first molar has the most complex developmental groove pattern of all the permanent mandibular molars. _____

39. The two roots of a permanent mandibular first molar are smaller, shorter, and less divergent than those of a second molar. _____

40. The pulp cavity of a permanent mandibular first molar is more likely to have three root canals—distal, mesiobuccal, and mesiolingual—and five pulp horns. _____

41. Permanent maxillary third molars, along with the mandibular third molars, commonly exhibit partial anodontia and thus are congenitally missing. _____

42. The defining oblique ridge is less prominent on the permanent maxillary second molar than on the first molar. _____

43. From the mesial, the mesial contact area of a permanent maxillary second molar is larger, and the cervical flattening or concavity is never as pronounced as in a first molar. _____

44. The two roots on permanent maxillary second molars are smaller than the first molars. _____

45. Loss of the tooth is followed by mesial inclination and drift of the maxillary second molar into the open arch space, and the mandibular first molar, if present, also supererupts. _____

46. On the permanent maxillary first molar, the two marginal ridges and two cusp ridges of the four major cusps are found bordering the occlusal table on the buccal and lingual margins. _____

47. The crown of any primary tooth is short in relation to its total length. _____

48. Overall, the dentin of the primary dentition is thicker than that of the permanent counterparts. _____

49. From the labial aspect, the crown of the primary maxillary central incisor appears wider mesiodistally than incisocervically, the opposite of its permanent successor. _____

50. The crown of the primary maxillary first molar does not resemble any other crown of either dentition. _____

Ordering

Place the following items in the correct order as indicated.

1. In what order should the following general dental terms be placed when giving the name of a tooth, going from the largest number of teeth included in an adult to the smallest number of teeth?

_____ a. Dentition

_____ b. Quadrant

_____ c. Arch

_____ d. Sextant

2. In what order should the following line angles of an anterior tooth be placed, going from mesial to distal for the front surface of the tooth and then in the same direction for the back surface of the tooth?

_____ a. Mesiolabial

_____ b. Distolabial

_____ c. Mesiolingual

_____ d. Distolingual

3. In what order should the following permanent incisors be placed, going from largest in overall size to smallest?

_____ a. Mandibular lateral

_____ b. Mandibular central

_____ c. Maxillary central

_____ d. Maxillary lateral

4. In what order should be following permanent teeth be placed according to their approximate eruption dates, going from earlier to later in time span?

_____ a. Mandibular central incisors

_____ b. Maxillary canines

_____ c. Maxillary first premolars

_____ d. Mandibular first molars

5. In what order should the following cusps of the permanent mandibular first molar be placed, going from largest in overall size to smallest?

_____ a. Mesiolingual

_____ b. Distolingual

_____ c. Distobuccal

_____ d. Mesiobuccal

6. In what order should the following cusps of the permanent maxillary first molar be placed, going from largest in overall size to smallest?

_____ a. Mesiolingual

_____ b. Distolingual

_____ c. Distobuccal

_____ d. Mesiobuccal

7. In what order should the following events during formation of the primary dentition be placed, going from earlier to later in time span?

_____ a. All teeth have started mineralization

_____ b. Beginning of tooth mineralization

_____ c. Completion of full dentition

_____ d. Eruption of first tooth into oral cavity

8. In what order should these skull features be placed, going from anterior to posterior on the skull?

_____ a. Postglenoid process

_____ b. Articular eminence

_____ c. Zygomatic arch

_____ d. Articular fossa

9. In what order should the following permanent premolars be placed, going from largest in overall size to smallest?

_____ a. Mandibular first

_____ b. Mandibular second

_____ c. Maxillary first

_____ d. Maxillary second

10. In what order should be following permanent teeth be placed according to their approximate eruption dates, going from earlier to later in time span?

_____ a. Maxillary lateral incisors

_____ b. Mandibular canines

_____ c. Maxillary second premolars

_____ d. Mandibular second molars

UNIT II: DENTAL EMBRYOLOGY CASE STUDY 1

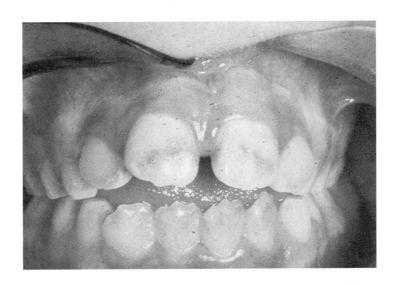

Patient	Female, 23 years old
Chief Complaint	*"Can we whiten my front teeth as soon as possible?"*
Background and/or Patient History	First-grade teacher Water fluoridation at naturally higher level as child Sucked thumb as child
Current Findings	New patient with regular 6-month dental care until recent move States teeth always stained with recommendation of full-coverage crowns when fully erupted Difficulty with homecare on small-sized teeth No fluoridated water now Regularly chews sugared gum

* Uses format of Integrated National Board Dental Examination by Joint Commission on National Dental Examinations by American Dental Association. Figures courtesy Margaret J. Fehrenbach, RDH, MS, unless otherwise noted.

1. What dental disturbance is present with the anterior teeth of both arches?
   A. Concrescence
   B. Enamel dysplasia
   C. Dentinal dysplasia
   D. Chronic pulpitis

2. Which of the following cell types were mainly disturbed so as to cause the chief complaint?
   A. Odontoblasts
   B. Fibroblasts
   C. Ameloblasts
   D. Cementoblasts

3. During which of the following stage(s) of odontogenesis does this dental disturbance of the anterior teeth occur?
   A. Bud stage
   B. Initiation stage
   C. Cap or bell stages
   D. Apposition and maturation stages

4. What is the exact type of staining present with the anterior teeth?
   A. Extrinsic
   B. Intrinsic
   C. Transient
   D. Temporary

5. Because of unusual bite noted with occlusion, what is also present on the masticatory surface of the mandibular anterior teeth?
   A. Attrition
   B. Perikymata
   C. Mamelons
   D. Occlusal tables

UNIT II: DENTAL EMBRYOLOGY CASE STUDY 2

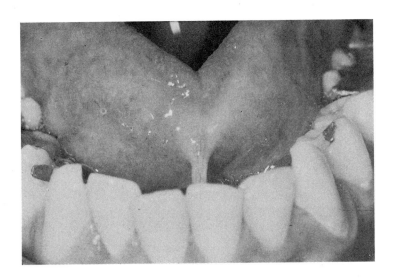

Patient	Male, 52 years old
Chief Complaint	*"My teeth on the lower jaw are getting more crowded."*
Background and/or Patient History	Historian at university Moderate speech impediment because never had suggested speech lessons, orofacial myofunctional therapy, or surgical procedures
Current Findings	New patient for initial examination Mandibular anterior teeth crowded with moderate lingual supragingival calculus

1. What orofacial disturbance is present?
   A. Gemination
   B. Fusion
   C. Ankyloglossia
   D. Cleft uvula

2. The orofacial disturbance mainly involves what part of the oral cavity?
   A. Lingual frenum
   B. Lingual gingiva
   C. Soft palate
   D. Soft tissue of tongue

3. In what week of prenatal development does the associated orofacial structure involved in the dental disturbance begin its specific development?
   A. First week
   B. Second week
   C. Third week
   D. Fourth week

4. Which of the following is the superficial demarcation of fusion noted in the associated structure(s) involved in this orofacial disturbance?
   A. Lateral lingual swellings
   B. Copula
   C. Epiglottic swelling
   D. Tuberculum impar

5. During what prenatal developmental time does the associated structure involved in the orofacial disturbance complete its fusion?
   A. Fetal period
   B. Embryonic period
   C. Initiation stage
   D. Maturation stage

UNIT II: DENTAL EMBRYOLOGY CASE STUDY 3

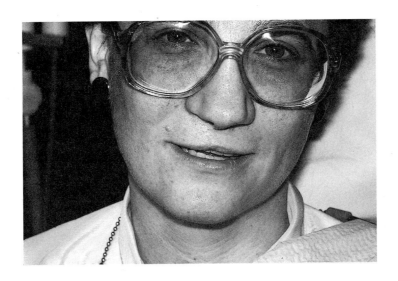

Patient	Female, 45 years old
Chief Complaint	*"Why do I have so much tartar on my teeth?"*
Background and/or Patient History	Surgery as child for birth defect that left a scar Speech lessons as child but still slight speech impediment Premenopausal Allergy to pollens Former smoker Medications: Decongestants Short-term hormone replacement therapy
Current Findings	New patient for initial examination No functional defects with mastication Mouth breather Maxillary anterior teeth with moderate facial inflammation Generalized moderate supragingival calculus Slight to moderate xerostomia with hyposalivation

1. Which of the following developmental disturbances was present?
   A. Fusion
   B. Cleft palate
   C. Cleft lip
   D. Spina bifida

2. Which of the following processes is mainly involved in the developmental disturbance?
   A. Maxillary process
   B. Lateral nasal process
   C. Mandibular process
   D. Frontonasal process

3. This developmental disturbance occurs more commonly and more severely in which of the following populations?
   A. Men
   B. Women
   C. Adolescent
   D. Geriatric

4. Which of the following statements is correct concerning this developmental disturbance?
   A. Only hereditary etiologic factors noted
   B. May be associated with other abnormalities
   C. Only occurs unilaterally
   D. Occurs mainly on right side

5. During which prenatal developmental time does this developmental disturbance occur?
   A. Preimplantation period
   B. Embryonic period
   C. Initiation stage
   D. Apposition stage

UNIT II: DENTAL EMBRYOLOGY CASE STUDY 4

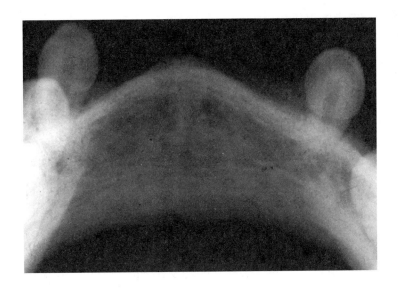

Patient	Male, 23 years of age
Chief Complaint	*"I need to know if I can have those implant teeth put in and when it can occur."*
Background and/or Patient History	Aspiring actor after finishing high school drama with honors Needs special measures to keep body temperature regulated Hearing difficulty due to genetic defect
Current Findings	New patient at community dental clinic referred by school nurse Looks older because of sparse hair Missing many teeth; wears ill-fitting upper and lower partial dentures Periodic partial dentures replaced over time since toddler States saving for dental implants placed through reduced-fee program at dental school An occlusal radiograph was taken of mandibular anterior sextant along with other radiographs

1. Which of the following developmental disturbances is present?
   A. Fetal alcohol syndrome
   B. Down syndrome
   C. Ectodermal dysplasia
   D. Spina bifida

2. Which of the following can be noted in this developmental disturbance case?
   A. Various levels of intellectual disability
   B. Indistinct philtrum and thin upper lip
   C. Abnormalities of skin, hair, and nails
   D. Epicanthic folds near eyes

3. The noted developmental disturbance has involvement with which of the following etiologic factors?
   A. Teratogenic
   B. Hereditary
   C. Radiation
   D. Drug usage

4. What of the following can be recommended for this case and would temporarily serve as both a cosmetic and functional purpose?
   A. Myofunctional therapy
   B. Replacement partial dentures
   C. Surgical removal of remaining teeth
   D. Monitored speech therapy

5. The structures involved with this developmental disturbance are formed during which prenatal developmental time?
   A. Fetal period
   B. Embryonic period
   C. Initiation stage
   D. Maturation stage

UNIT II: DENTAL EMBRYOLOGY CASE STUDY 5

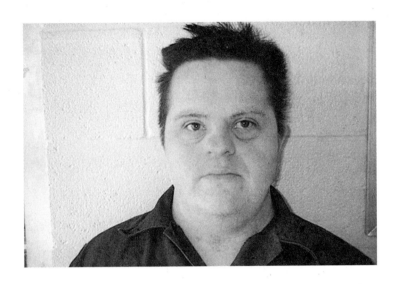

Patient	Male, 26 years of age
Chief Complaint	*"I need teeth done."*
Background and/or Patient History	Group home after being home schooled Works part time at library Hypothyroidism related to genetic disturbance Sleep apnea Past speech therapy Medications: Thyroid hormone Antiseizure medication
Current Findings	Current patient of record for 6-month appointment examination Microdontia with short conical roots Undersized jawbone structure Chronic periodontal disease with moderate early bone loss Xerostomia Mouth breather

1. Which of the following developmental disturbances is present?
   A. Fetal alcohol syndrome
   B. Down syndrome
   C. Ectodermal dysplasia
   D. Spina bifida

2. During what prenatal developmental event does this disturbance occur?
   A. Meiosis
   B. Mitosis
   C. Maturation stage
   D. Mesoderm formation

3. What situation was mainly involved during this developmental disturbance?
   A. Ectopic pregnancy
   B. Infective teratogen
   C. Trisomy 21
   D. Neural tube defect

4. Which of the following may also be present?
   A. Fissures of the tongue
   B. Enlarged tongue
   C. Hyperplasia of lingual papillae
   D. Furrowed upper lip

5. Which of the following is the correct number of chromosomes present after the joining of the sperm and ovum but that may not have occurred with this fertilization?
   A. 12
   B. 23
   C. 46
   D. 92

UNIT II: DENTAL EMBRYOLOGY CASE STUDY 6*

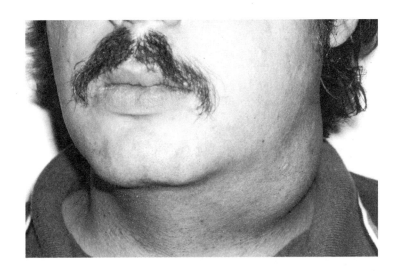

Patient	Male, 32 years of age
Chief Complaint	*"What is the swelling here on my neck?"*
Background and/or Patient History	Business administrator who wants a diagnosis before entering new job position Allergy to pollen OTC allergy medications No history of night sweats, unexplained weight loss, or chronic fatigue
Current Findings	New patient limited examination Large soft swelling on left side of neck near angle of mandible States that lesion present over 2 years; lesion slowly growing larger No red skin patches noted over lesion No fever or soreness noted upon palpation of neck lesion Wave effect felt upon palpation of neck lesion

* Figure from Neville BW, et al.: *Oral and Maxillofacial Pathology,* 4th ed., St. Louis, Elsevier, 2016.

1. Which of the following is the most likely diagnosis for the neck enlargement?
    A. Lymph node infection
    B. Thyroid gland goiter
    C. Temporomandibular disorder
    D. Branchial cleft cyst

2. Why does this lesion occur in this region of the neck?
    A. Transformation of branchial or pharyngeal apparatus
    B. Serious infection of regional primary lymph nodes
    C. Secondary pain impulses from nearby joint
    D. Growth from surge in specific hormones

3. Which of the following usually occurs during the development of the thyroid gland?
    A. Foramen cecum shows origin of thyroid gland
    B. Migration of gland into the jaw region
    C. Foramen cecum opens up to become persistent
    D. Cystic formation near sulcus terminalis

4. What occurs during the development of branchial or pharyngeal apparatus?
    A. Tuberculum impar does not disappear during formation
    B. Area branchial or pharyngeal grooves are not obliterated
    C. First two arch pairs develop to greatest extent
    D. Migration pathway of thyroid gland into region

5. Which of the following is present with gross biopsy of healthy lymph nodes with lesion removal?
    A. Germinal centers containing mature lymphocytes
    B. Budding of nearby blood vessels into nodular region
    C. Hilus at depression on one side of node
    D. Presence of multiple efferent vessels

UNIT III: DENTAL HISTOLOGY CASE STUDY 1

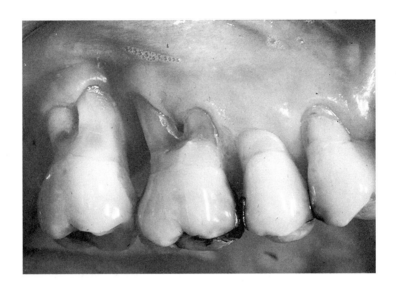

Patient	Female, 57 years of age
Chief Complaint	*"Why do my teeth look so long lately and are also so loose?"*
Background and/or Patient History	Retired tennis player History of skin cancer Diagnosed with chronic periodontal disease
Current Findings	New patient with regular dental care until 15 years ago when dentist retired Generalized exposed roots with moderate to severe bone loss Generalized slight bleeding and moderate mobility

1. What part of the alveolar process has the patient lost between the roots of the molars?
   A. Basal bone
   B. Alveolar crest bone
   C. Interdental septum
   D. Interradicular septum

2. What fiber group of the periodontal ligament is the last group to be affected by periodontal disease?
   A. Alveolar crest group
   B. Horizontal group
   C. Oblique group
   D. Interdental group

3. Both the patient's lost alveolar process and altered periodontal ligament are considered part of which of the following orofacial structures?
   A. Periodontium
   B. Alveolodental ligament
   C. Principal fiber groups
   D. Temporomandibular joint

4. What part of each of the posterior teeth was first lost as a result of the root exposure?
   A. Predentin
   B. Secondary dentin
   C. Cellular cementum
   D. Coronal enamel

5. Which cell population has been most active in removing the alveolar process because of the chronic periodontal disease?
   A. Ameloblast
   B. Osteoclast
   C. Odontoblast
   D. Odontoclast

UNIT III: DENTAL HISTOLOGY CASE STUDY 2

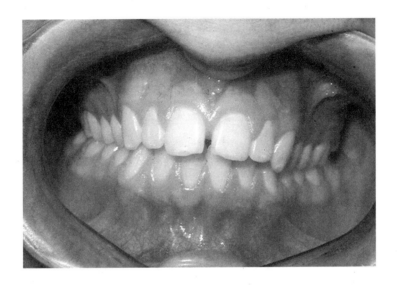

Patient	Male, 32 years of age
Chief Complaint	*"Why do my teeth keep bleeding when I floss?"*
Background and/or Patient History	Real estate agent with four children Height: 5 feet, 11 inches (1.80 metres) Weight: 280 pounds (127 kilograms) BP: 110/85 Diabetes mellitus type 2 Medication: Oral diabetes pill States does not routinely take medication or test blood since job setback
Current Findings	Generalized moderate bleeding No bone loss on radiographs Previous dental office recommended brushing teeth more Does not regularly brush or floss

1. What type of mucosa is involved in the inflammation noted?
   A. Lining mucosa
   B. Specialized mucosa
   C. Masticatory mucosa
   D. Paranasal mucosa

2. Which fiber group associated with the periodontal ligament is the first group to be affected with the patient's inflammation?
   A. Gingival group
   B. Alveolar crest group
   C. Horizontal group
   D. Oblique group

3. What is the main underlying cause of the gingival bleeding when flossing?
   A. Thickening of the junctional epithelium
   B. Repair of the lamina propria's blood vessels
   C. Increased blood vessels in the lamina propria
   D. Increased collagen production around blood vessels

4. What is the exact term used when dealing with the present periodontal condition?
   A. Active gingivitis
   B. Chronic gingivitis
   C. Active periodontitis
   D. Chronic periodontitis

5. What histologic situation is present in both the epithelium and lamina propria at the dentogingival junction?
   A. Smooth interface at basement membrane between tissue types
   B. Decreased numbers of migrating white blood cells
   C. Formation of rete pegs and connective tissue papillae
   D. All signs of chronic inflammation throughout tissue types

UNIT III: DENTAL HISTOLOGY CASE STUDY 3

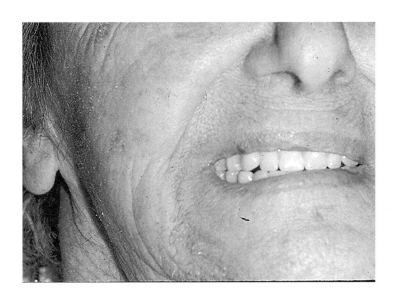

Patient	Female, 82 years of age
Chief Complaint	*"My mouth feels dry."*
Background and/or Patient History	Extended care facility resident Alzheimer disease early stages Medication: Antidepressant Former smoker
Current Findings	New patient at limited facility dental clinic Moderate level of dry mouth Complete dentures do not fit comfortably

1. What is the term used to describe the dry mouth condition present?
   A. Erosion
   B. Abfraction
   C. Hyposalivation
   D. Xerostomia

2. Which is the largest salivary gland present?
   A. Parotid
   B. Submandibular
   C. Sublingual
   D. von Ebner

3. What salivary gland usually produces the most saliva in the oral cavity?
   A. Parotid
   B. Submandibular
   C. Sublingual
   D. von Ebner

4. What part of each of the jaws is still completely present?
   A. Basal bone
   B. Alveolar process
   C. Interdental septum
   D. Interradicular septum

5. What is the diminished length of the lower third of the face termed?
   A. Increase in facial Golden Proportions
   B. Loss of vertical dimension
   C. Partially edentulous state
   D. Mesial drift with super-eruption

UNIT III: DENTAL HISTOLOGY CASE STUDY 4

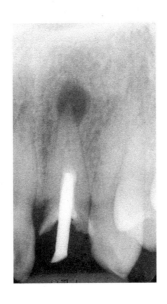

Patient	Male, 45 years of age
Chief Complaint	*"Can you fix my painful broken tooth?"*
Background and/or Patient History	High school basketball coach States tooth had endodontic therapy in twenties by referred specialist due to dental anomaly No longer chews spit tobacco
Current Findings	Patient of record with limited examination Broken anterior tooth Pain on percussion when chewing on tooth Has bad taste in mouth

1. What is the dental anomaly that was present in this tooth?
   A. Fusion
   B. Gemination
   C. Dens in dente
   D. Peg lateral

2. Why is there pain with this tooth?
   A. Secondary dentin filling pulp chamber
   B. Inflammatory edema pressing on nerves
   C. Inert material extruding from the pulp
   D. Apical bone forming at the apex

3. What is the best explanation for the tooth breaking?
   A. Darkening of the tooth
   B. Failure during lobular division
   C. Loss of tooth vitality
   D. Placement of gutta-percha

4. What is the main path by which pulpal infection travels to the surrounding apical periodontium to cause an abscess?
   A. Apical foramen
   B. Pulp horns
   C. Accessory canals
   D. Dentinal tubules

5. Which of the following cell populations can produce additional pulp tissue after an injury such as the one experienced?
   A. Odontoblasts
   B. Red blood cells
   C. White blood cells
   D. Undifferentiated mesenchymal cells

UNIT III: DENTAL HISTOLOGY
CASE STUDY 5

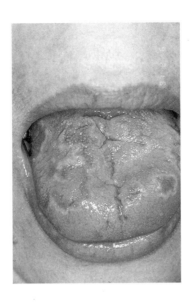

Patient	Female, 32 years of age
Chief Complaint	*"Why does the top of my tongue always look funny?"*
Background and/or Patient History	Chef in restaurant Recent emigrant with excellent past dental care Osteoporosis Takes calcium supplement States tongue has always looked this way
Current Findings	Second visit at dental school clinic after screening for complete examination Uses electric toothbrush since recommended at last visit Brushes dorsal surface of tongue regularly

1. What is the condition noted on the dorsal surface of the tongue?
   A. Fissured tongue
   B. Central papillary atrophy
   C. Geographic tongue
   D. Burning mouth syndrome

2. What type of lingual papillae is mainly involved in this tongue condition?
   A. Filiform
   B. Fungiform
   C. Circumvallate
   D. Foliate

3. What type of oral mucosa is mainly associated with this condition on the dorsal surface of the tongue?
   A. Masticatory
   B. Lining
   C. Specialized
   D. Paranasal

4. Which of the following is associated with sensory neuron processes when the patient is working?
   A. Taste pore
   B. Taste cells
   C. Supporting cells
   D. Surrounding tongue epithelium

5. What area of the tongue has never had any fungiform lingual papillae present?
   A. Sulcus terminalis
   B. Tip of the tongue
   C. Body of the tongue
   D. Near filiform lingual papillae

UNIT III: DENTAL HISTOLOGY
CASE STUDY 6

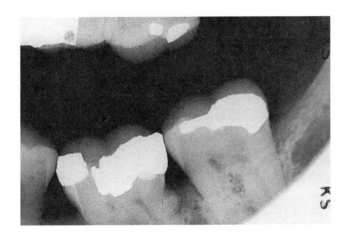

Patient	Female, 34 years of age
Chief Complaint	*"There are bumps on the sides of my lower molars when I floss."*
Background and/or Patient History	Student nurse Diabetes mellitus type 1 Medication: Insulin injections twice daily
Current Findings	New patient limited examination Single radiograph of areas of concern Generalized slight bleeding upon periodontal probing of certain posterior teeth but no calculus noted in these areas Just started flossing teeth

1. What could be causing the situation with the molars noted?
   A. Denticles
   B. Enamel pearls
   C. Cemental spurs
   D. Cementicles

2. What does this noted situation with the molars involve?
   A. Deposition by misplaced ameloblasts
   B. Irregular deposition by cementocytes
   C. Apposition around cellular debris
   D. Calcified masses of dentin

3. What is the main histologic tissue associated with this situation with the molars?
   A. Cementoblasts
   B. Dentinal tubules
   C. Enamel rods
   D. Fibroblasts

4. Which of the following is important to stress to maintain oral health?
   A. Avoidance of flossing
   B. Taking medication as prescribed
   C. Avoiding radiographic examinations
   D. Rinsing with salt water

5. Which dental procedures of the following need to be completed at this appointment?
   A. Scaling off of involved areas
   B. Removal by pumice
   C. Nutritional counseling
   D. Periodic radiographic examination

UNIT IV: DENTAL ANATOMY
CASE STUDY 1

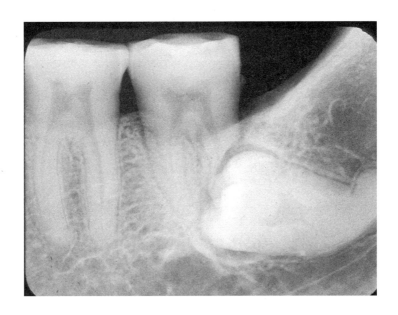

Patient	Male, 25 years of age
Chief Complaint	*"Why does my lower jaw hurt even when using my guard?"*
Background and/or Patient History	Chemistry postgraduate student Orthodontic therapy 10 years ago at referred orthodontic office States uses nightguard regularly
Current Findings	Patient of record with low caries risk Moderate level of bruxism Generalized moderate attrition Early symptoms of jaw joint disorder Painful area in lower left jaw but no lesions present

1. What is the condition noted on the radiograph that is probably causing oral pain?
   A. Cyst formation
   B. Microdontia
   C. Partial anodontia
   D. Impacted third molar

2. Which of the following are features of the tooth that is causing the discomfort?
   A. Three roots
   B. Four pulp horns
   C. Consistent crown form
   D. Square crown outline

3. When does this tooth usually complete its roots?
   A. 10 to 14 years
   B. 13 to 17 years
   C. 17 to 21 years
   D. 18 to 25 years

4. What are the opaque structures noted in the pulp chambers of some of the mandibular posterior teeth?
   A. Denticles
   B. Pulp stones
   C. Sialoliths
   D. Enamel pearls

5. Which structure is located on the temporal bone anterior to the articular fossa of the jaw joint?
   A. Joint capsule
   B. Articular eminence
   C. Synovial membrane
   D. Articulating surface of the condyle

UNIT IV: DENTAL ANATOMY
CASE STUDY 2

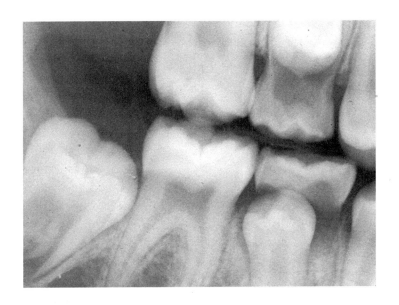

Patient	Male, 11 years of age
Chief Complaint	*"Why do my back teeth feel real loose when I wiggle them?"*
Background and/or Patient History	Likes to play basketball Drinks soft drinks regularly
Current Findings	Patient of record annual examination Enamel sealants placed last appointment Four posterior teeth are loose with another four teeth partially erupted with tissue inflamed

1. On which teeth were enamel sealants probably placed at last dental appointment?
   A. First premolars
   B. Second premolars
   C. First molars
   D. Second molars

2. Which partially erupted teeth may require placement of enamel sealants at the next appointment because of increased risk of caries?
   A. First premolars
   B. Second premolars
   C. First molars
   D. Second molars

3. Which of the following teeth may be loose and ready to be exfoliated?
   A. S
   B. T
   C. #2
   D. #30

4. The crown of which posterior tooth appears similar to the crown anatomy of one of the nearby loose teeth?
   A. S
   B. T
   C. #2
   D. #30

5. Which of the following teeth may have already been exfoliated?
   A. S
   B. T
   C. #2
   D. #30

UNIT IV: DENTAL ANATOMY
CASE STUDY 3

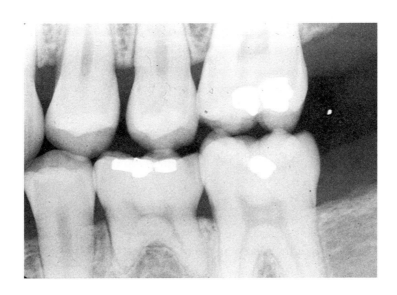

Patient	Female, 25 years of age
Chief Complaint	*"Why is one of my back teeth on each side smaller than the rest?"*
Background and/or Patient History	Sealants placed at age 6 but later restored due to margin failure Four permanent posterior teeth extracted at age 13 because of extensive caries Four teeth extracted age 20 because of impaction Last dentist said some "adult" teeth were never going to erupt Does not have fluoridated water
Current Findings	New patient initial examination Smaller bilateral mandibular posterior teeth Difficulty with homecare on smaller-sized teeth Regularly chews sugared gum

1. Which permanent posterior teeth exhibit partial anodontia?
   A. Second premolars
   B. First molars
   C. Second molars
   D. Third molars

2. Which permanent posterior teeth were extracted as an adolescent?
   A. Second premolars
   B. First molars
   C. Second molars
   D. Third molars

3. Which permanent posterior teeth were extracted as a young adult?
   A. Second premolars
   B. First molars
   C. Second molars
   D. Third molars

4. Which permanent posterior teeth have been restored because of failure of the enamel sealants?
   A. Second premolars
   B. First molars
   C. Second molars
   D. Third molars

5. Of the teeth now present, which of the following mandibular teeth have two roots?
   A. Second premolars
   B. First molars
   C. Second molars
   D. Third molars

UNIT IV: DENTAL ANATOMY CASE STUDY 4

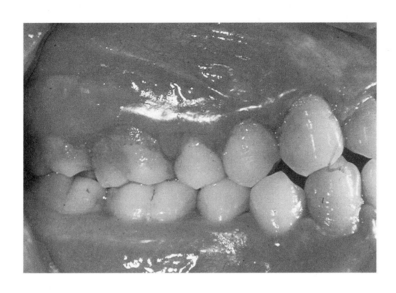

Patient	Male, 42 years of age
Chief Complaint	*"Why are my bottom eyeteeth sensitive at the gumline when I drink fresh coffee?"*
Background and/or Patient History	Height: 5 feet, 10 inches (1.78 metres) Weight: 180 pounds (81.6 kilograms) BP: 115/95 High blood pressure controlled with medication Medication: Diuretic Former smoker Orthodontic therapy 25 years ago but does not have any form of retention Extracted permanent third molars at age 20 Not been to dental office for 12 years States grinding teeth at night
Current Findings	Very nervous new patient for initial examination No caries Generalized moderate gingival inflammation with generalized soft deposits Uses soft toothbrush Gargles with OTC medicated mouthrinses

1. What is the correct angle classification of malocclusion on posterior dentition on the right side?
   A. Class I
   B. Class II, Division I
   C. Class II, Division II
   D. Class III

2. What other occlusal evaluation notes can be made regarding the right side of the dentition?
   A. Severe crossbite
   B. Open bite
   C. Severe overjet
   D. End-to-end bite

3. What may be occurring on the mandibular teeth to make them sensitive to hot fluids?
   A. Erosion
   B. Abfraction
   C. Pulpitis
   D. Toothbrush abrasion

4. What is the correct term used for this nighttime habit with the teeth?
   A. Clenching
   B. Xerostomia
   C. Bruxism
   D. Passive eruption

5. What part of the anatomy of each sensitive tooth is first lost with grinding?
   A. Fossae
   B. Pits
   C. Grooves
   D. Cusps

UNIT IV: DENTAL ANATOMY
CASE STUDY 5*

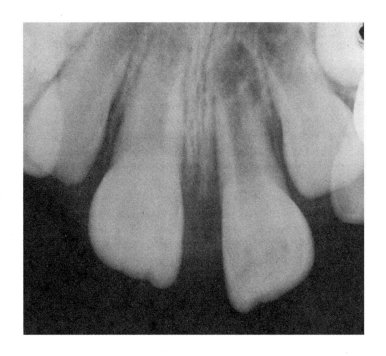

Patient	Male, 7 years of age
Chief Complaint	Mother: *"My son's front tooth looks different now!"*
Background and/or Patient History	Patient of record mother states he slipped in tub and hit upper front tooth 20 minutes earlier No medical concerns
Current Findings	Patient of record emergency appointment Generalized slight bleeding in front of upper mouth Swollen upper lip No other acute or chronic trauma noted and negative for concussion Periapical radiograph taken of involved tooth

* Figure from Dean JA: *McDonald and Avery's Dentistry for the Child and Adolescent*, 10th ed., St. Louis, Mosby/Elsevier, 2016.

1. What dentition period is present and with how many teeth?
   A. Deciduous dentition period, 10 teeth
   B. Primary dentition period, 20 teeth
   C. Mixed dentition period, 24 teeth
   D. Transitional dentition period, 30 teeth

2. Which of the following teeth should be fully erupted?
   A. Incisors, canines, first molars
   B. Incisors, canines, molars
   C. Incisors, canines, premolars
   D. Incisors, canines, premolars, molars

3. What effect might this accident have on the future development of the injured tooth?
   A. Pulpal involvement
   B. Slight crown shortening
   C. Additional primary dentin layers
   D. None anticipated

4. When does the root commonly complete its development for the involved tooth?
   A. Age 6
   B. Age 7
   C. Age 10
   D. Age 12

5. Which of the following is an anatomic attribute of the involved tooth?
   A. Nonsuccedaneous tooth
   B. Distal contact at middle third
   C. Wider labiolingually than mesiodistally
   D. Labial and lingual height of contour in cervical third

Notes

Notes

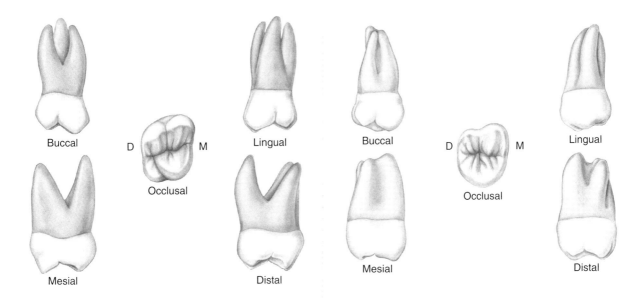

Buccal

D Occlusal M

Lingual

Mesial

Distal

Buccal

D Occlusal M

Lingual

Mesial

Distal

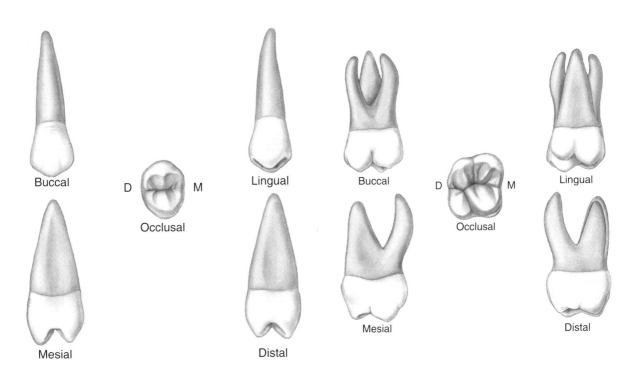

Buccal

D Occlusal M

Lingual

Mesial

Distal

Buccal

D Occlusal M

Lingual

Mesial

Distal

Maxillary Right Third Molar (Heart-shaped Occlusal Outline)

CHARACTERISTICS:

Universal Number: #1 **International Number:** #18
Eruption: 17-21
Root completion: 18-25
General crown features: Occlusal table with marginal ridges and cusps with tips, inclined planes, ridges, grooves, fossae, pits
Specific crown features: Smaller crown than second and variable in form. Heart-shaped or rhomboidal crown outline with three or four cusps. Buccal cervical ridge
Height of Contour: Buccal: cervical third; Lingual: middle third
Mesial contact: Middle third
Distal contact: None
Distinguishing right from left: Distobuccal cusp shorter than mesiobuccal cusp. Roots curve distally
General Root Features: Three roots
Specific Root features: Less divergent roots. Usually fused roots. Roots curving distally

Maxillary Right Second Molar (Rhomboidal Crown Outline)

CHARACTERISTICS:

Universal Number: #2 **International Number:** #17
Eruption: 12-13
Root completion: 14-16
General crown features: Occlusal table with marginal ridges and cusps with tips, inclined planes, ridges, grooves, fossae, pits
Specific crown features: Smaller crown than first. Heart-shaped or rhomboidal crown outline, with three or four cusps. Less prominent oblique ridge. Mesiobuccal cusp longer than distobuccal cusp. Distolingual cusp smaller than on first or absent. No fifth cusp. Buccal cervical ridge
Height of Contour: Buccal: cervical third; Lingual: middle third
Mesial contact: Middle third
Distal contact: Middle third
Distinguishing right from left: Mesiolingual cusp outline longer and larger but not as sharp as distolingual cusp outline
General Root features: Three roots
Specific Root Features: Furcations. Root trunks and root concavities. Less divergent roots

Maxillary Right First Molar

CHARACTERISTICS:

Universal Number: #3 **International Number:** #16
Eruption: 6-7
Root completion: 9-10
General crown features: Occlusal table with marginal ridges and cusps with tips, inclined planes, ridges, grooves, fossae, and pits
Specific crown features: Largest tooth in arch and largest crown in dentition. Prominent oblique ridge. Four major cusps with buccal cusps almost equal in height. Fifth minor cusp of Carabelli associated with mesiolingual cusp. Buccal cervical ridge
Height of Contour: Buccal: cervical third; Lingual: middle third
Mesial contact: Junction of occlusal and middle thirds
Distal contact: Middle third
Distinguishing right from left: Mesiolingual cusp outline longer and larger but not as sharp as distolingual cusp outline
General Root features: Three roots
Specific Root Features: Furcations well removed from CEJ. Root trunks and root concavities. Divergent roots

Maxillary Right Second Premolar

CHARACTERISTICS:

Universal Number: #4 **International Number:** #15
Eruption: 10-12
Root completion: 12-14
General crown features: Occlusal table with marginal ridges and cusps with tips, ridges, inclined planes, grooves, fossae, pits
Specific crown features: Smaller than first. Two cusps same length. Short central groove with increased supplemental grooves. No mesial surface features like first. Buccal ridge
Height of Contour: Buccal: cervical third; Lingual: middle third
Mesial contact: Just cervical to junction of occlusal and middle thirds
Distal contact: Just cervical to junction of occlusal and middle thirds
Distinguishing right from left: Lingual cusp to offset to mesial
General root features: Single root
Specific root features: Elliptical on cervical cross section. Proximal root concavities

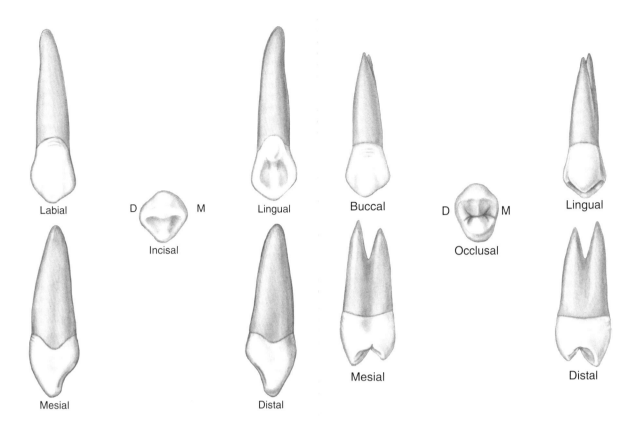

Labial — D / M — Incisal — Lingual

Mesial — Distal

Buccal — D / M — Occlusal — Lingual

Mesial — Distal

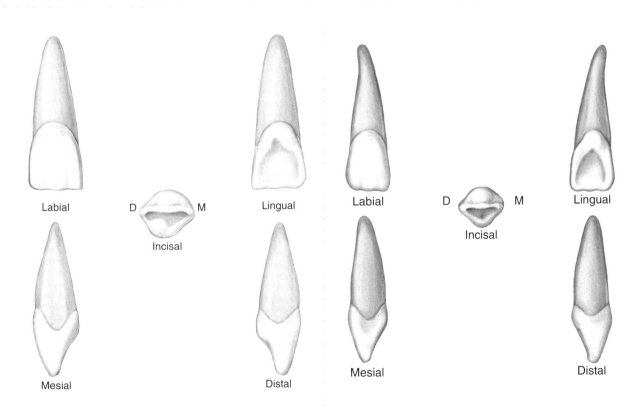

Labial — D / M — Incisal — Lingual

Mesial — Distal

Labial — D / M — Incisal — Lingual

Mesial — Distal

Maxillary Right First Premolar

CHARACTERISTICS:

Universal Number: #5 **International Number:** #14
Eruption 10-11
Root completion: 12-13
General crown features: Occlusal table with marginal ridges and cusps with tips, ridges, inclined planes, grooves, fossae, pits
Specific crown features: Larger than second. Buccal cusp longer of two cusps. Long central groove. Mesial surface features unlike second. Buccal ridge
Height of Contour: Buccal: cervical third; Lingual: middle third
Mesial contact: Just cervical to junction of occlusal and middle thirds
Distal contact: Just cervical to junction of occlusal and middle thirds
Distinguishing right from left: Longer mesial cusp slope than distal cusp slope and with mesial features: deeper CEJ curvature, marginal groove, developmental depression
General root features: Two roots with root trunk
Specific root features: Elliptical on cervical cross section. Proximal root concavities

Maxillary Right Canine

CHARACTERISTICS:

Universal Number: #6 **International Number:** #13
Eruption: 11-12
Root completion: 13-15
General crown features: Single cusp with tip, slopes, labial ridge, cingulum, lingual ridge, marginal ridges, lingual fossae
Specific crown features: Longest tooth in arch. Prominent lingual surface. Sharp cusp tip
Height of contour: Labial: cervical third; Lingual: middle third
Mesial contact: Junction of incisal third and middle thirds
Distal contact: Middle third
Distinguishing right from left: Shorter mesial cusp slope than distal cusp slope with more pronounced mesial CEJ curvature. More cervical contact on distal. Shorter distal outline than mesial outline on labial view and with depression between distal contact and CEJ
General root features: Long, thick single root
Specific root features: Oval on cervical cross section. Proximal root concavities. Blunt root apex

Maxillary Right Lateral Incisor

CHARACTERISTICS:

Universal Number: #7 **International Number:** #12
Eruption: 8-9
Root completion: 11
General crown features: Incisal ridge, incisal angles, cingulum, marginal ridges, lingual fossa
Specific crown features: Greatest crown variation. Like smaller central. Pronounced lingual surface with centered cingulum and prominent marginal ridges
Height of contour: Cervical third
Mesial contact: Incisal third
Distal contact: Middle third
Distinguishing right from left: Sharper mesioincisal angle and rounder distoincisal angle. More pronounced mesial CEJ curvature
General root features: Single root
Specific root features: Oval on cervical cross section. Same or longer than central but thinner. Overall conical shape. No proximal root concavities. Root curves distally with sharp apex

Maxillary Right Central Incisor

CHARACTERISTICS:

Universal Number: #8 **International Number:** #11
Eruption: 7-8
Root completion: 10
General crown features: Incisal ridge, incisal angles, cingulum, marginal ridges, lingual fossa
Specific crown features: Widest crown mesiodistally. Greatest CEJ curve and height of contour. Pronounced distal offset cingulum and marginal ridges with wide and deep lingual fossa
Height of contour: Cervical third
Mesial contact: Incisal third
Distal contact: Junction of incisal and middle thirds
Distinguishing right from left: Sharper mesioincisal angle and rounder distoincisal angle. More pronounced mesial CEJ curvature
General root features: Single root
Specific root features: Triangular on cervical cross section. Overall conical shape. No proximal root concavities. Rounded apex

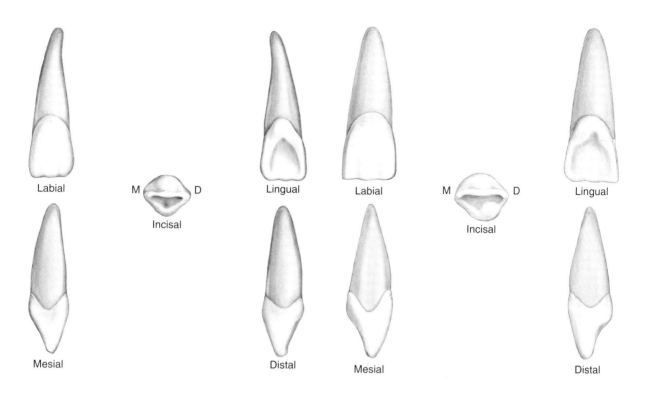

Labial

M ⊕ D
Incisal

Lingual

Mesial

Distal

Labial

M ⊕ D
Incisal

Lingual

Mesial

Distal

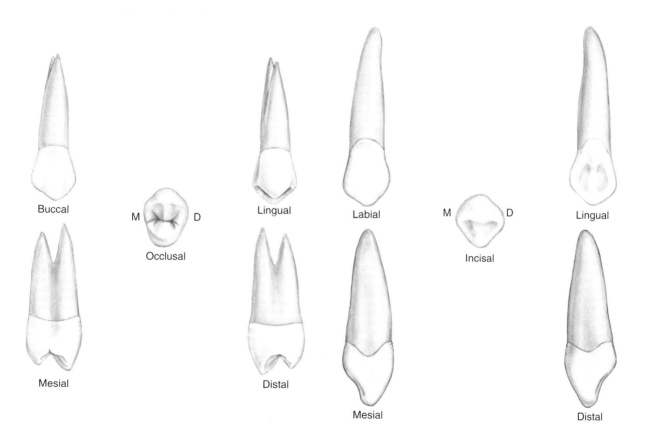

Buccal

M ⊕ D
Occlusal

Lingual

Mesial

Distal

Labial

M ⊕ D
Incisal

Lingual

Mesial

Distal

Maxillary Left Central Incisor

CHARACTERISTICS:

Universal Number: #9 **International Number:** #21
Eruption: 7-8
Root completion: 10
General crown features: Incisal ridge, incisal angles, cingulum, marginal ridges, lingual fossa
Specific crown features: Widest crown mesiodistally. Greatest CEJ curve and height of contour. Pronounced distal offset cingulum and marginal ridges with wide and deep lingual fossa
Height of contour: Cervical third
Mesial contact: Incisal third
Distal contact: Junction of incisal and middle thirds
Distinguishing right from left: Sharper mesioincisal angle and rounder distoincisal angle. More pronounced mesial CEJ curvature
General root features: Single root
Specific root features: Triangular on cervical cross section. Overall conical shape. No proximal root concavities. Rounded apex

Maxillary Left Lateral Incisor

CHARACTERISTICS:

Universal Number: #10 **International Number:** #22
Eruption: 8-9
Root completion: 11
General crown features: Incisal ridge, incisal angles, cingulum, marginal ridges, lingual fossa
Specific crown features: Greatest crown variation. Like smaller central. Pronounced lingual surface with centered cingulum and prominent marginal ridges
Height of contour: Cervical third
Mesial contact: Incisal third
Distal contact: Middle third
Distinguishing right from left: Sharper mesioincisal angle and rounder distoincisal angle. More pronounced mesial CEJ curvature
General root features: Single root
Specific root features: Oval on cervical cross section. Same or longer than central but thinner. Overall conical shape. No proximal root concavities. Root curves distally with sharp apex

Maxillary Left Canine

CHARACTERISTICS:

Universal Number: #11 **International Number:** #23
Eruption: 11-12
Root completion: 13-15
General crown features: Single cusp with tip, slopes, labial ridge, cingulum, lingual ridge, marginal ridges, lingual fossae
Specific crown features: Longest tooth in arch. Prominent lingual surface. Sharp cusp tip
Height of contour: Labial: cervical third; Lingual: middle third
Mesial contact: Junction of incisal third and middle thirds
Distal contact: Middle third
Distinguishing right from left: Shorter mesial cusp slope than distal cusp slope, with more pronounced mesial CEJ curvature. More cervical contact on distal. Shorter distal outline than mesial outline on labial view and with depression between distal contact and CEJ
General root features: Long, thick single root
Specific root features: Oval on cervical cross section. Proximal root concavities. Blunt root apex

Maxillary Left First Premolar

CHARACTERISTICS:

Universal Number: #12 **International Number:** #24
Eruption: 10-11
Root completion: 12-13
General crown features: Occlusal table with marginal ridges and cusps and with tips, ridges, inclined planes, grooves, fossae, pits
Specific crown features: Larger than second. Buccal cusp longer of two cusps. Long central groove. Mesial surface features unlike second. Buccal ridge
Height of Contour: Buccal: cervical third; Lingual: middle third
Mesial contact: Just cervical to junction of occlusal and middle thirds
Distal contact: Just cervical to junction of occlusal and middle thirds
Distinguishing right from left: Longer mesial cusp slope than distal cusp slope, with mesial **features:** deeper CEJ curvature, marginal groove, developmental depression
General root features: Two roots with root trunk
Specific root features: Elliptical on cervical cross section. Proximal root concavities

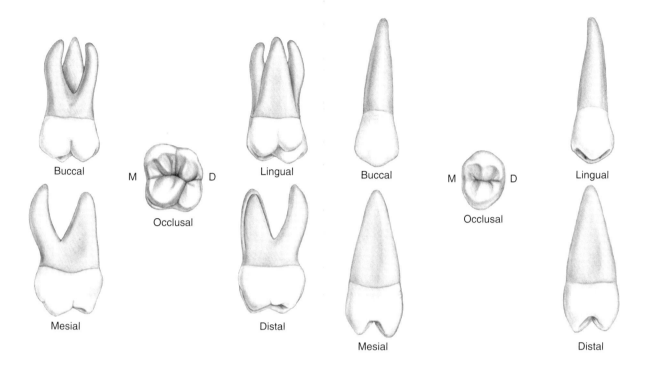

Buccal
M Occlusal D
Lingual
Mesial
Distal

Buccal
M Occlusal D
Lingual
Mesial
Distal

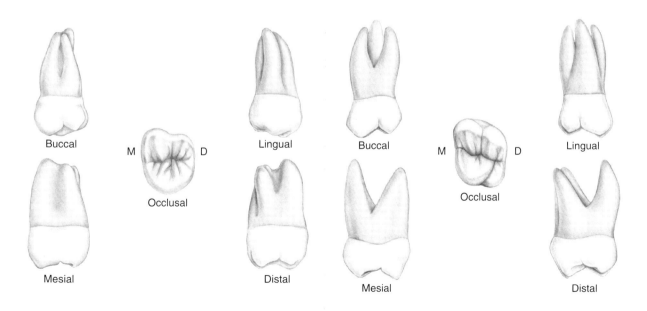

Buccal
M Occlusal D
Lingual
Mesial
Distal

Buccal
M Occlusal D
Lingual
Mesial
Distal

Maxillary Left Second Premolar

CHARACTERISTICS:

Universal Number: #13 **International Number:** #25
Eruption: 10-12
Root completion: 12-14
General crown features: Occlusal table with marginal ridges and cusps with tips, ridges, inclined planes, grooves, fossae, pits
Specific crown features: Smaller than first. Two cusps same length. Short central groove with increased supplemental grooves. No mesial surface features like first. Buccal ridge
Height of Contour: Buccal: cervical third; Lingual: middle third
Mesial contact: Just cervical to junction of occlusal and middle thirds
Distal contact: Just cervical to junction of occlusal and middle thirds
Distinguishing right from left: Lingual cusp to offset to mesial
General root features: Single root
Specific root features: Elliptical on cervical cross section. Proximal root concavities

Maxillary Left First Molar

CHARACTERISTICS:

Universal Number: #14 **International Number:** #26
Eruption: 6-7
Root completion: 9-10
General crown features: Occlusal table with marginal ridges and cusps with tips, inclined planes, ridges, grooves, fossae, and pits. Buccal cervical ridge
Specific crown features: Largest tooth in arch, largest crown in dentition. Four major cusps, with buccal cusps almost equal in height. Fifth minor cusp of Carabelli associated with mesiolingual cusp and prominent oblique ridge
Height of Contour: Buccal: cervical third; Lingual: middle third
Mesial contact: Junction of occlusal and middle thirds
Distal contact: Middle third
Distinguishing right from left: Mesiolingual cusp outline longer and larger but not as sharp as distolingual cusp outline
General Root features: Three roots
Specific Root Features: Furcations well removed from CEJ. Root trunks and root concavities. Divergent roots

Maxillary Left Second Molar (Rhomboidal Crown Outline)

CHARACTERISTICS:

Universal Number: #15 **International Number:** #27
Eruption: 12-13
Root completion: 14-16
General crown features: Occlusal table with marginal ridges and cusps with tips, inclined planes, ridges, grooves, fossae, and pits
Specific crown features: Smaller crown than first. Heart-shaped or rhomboidal crown outline, with three or four cusps. Less prominent oblique ridge. Mesiobuccal cusp longer than distobuccal cusp. Distolingual cusp smaller than on first or absent. No fifth cusp. Buccal cervical ridge
Height of Contour: Buccal: cervical third; Lingual: middle third
Mesial contact: Middle third
Distal contact: Middle third
Distinguishing right from left: Mesiolingual cusp outline longer and larger but not as sharp as distolingual cusp outline
General Root features: Three roots
Specific Root Features: Furcations. Root trunks and root concavities. Less divergent roots

Maxillary Left Third Molar (Heart-shaped Occlusal Outline)

CHARACTERISTICS:

Universal Number: #16 **International Number:** #28
Eruption: 17-21
Root completion: 18-25
General crown features: Occlusal table with marginal ridges and cusps with tips, inclined planes, ridges, grooves, fossae, and pits
Specific crown features: Smaller crown than second and variable in form. Heart-shaped or rhomboidal crown outline, with three or four cusps. Buccal cervical ridge
Height of Contour: Buccal: cervical third; Lingual: middle third
Mesial contact: Middle third
Distal contact: None
Distinguishing right from left: Distobuccal cusp shorter than mesiobuccal cusp. Roots curve distally
General Root Features: Three roots
Specific Root features: Less divergent roots. Usually fused roots, curving distally

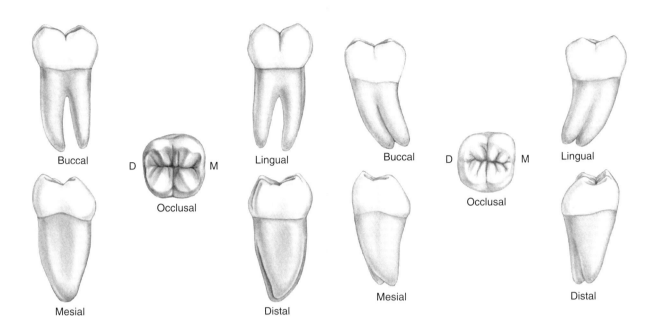

Buccal

D Occlusal M

Lingual

Mesial

Distal

Buccal

D Occlusal M

Lingual

Mesial

Distal

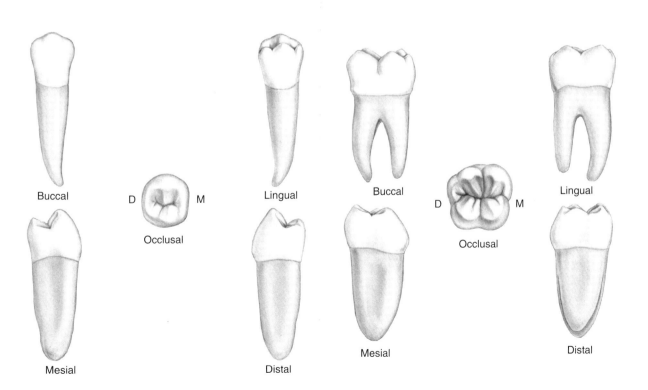

Buccal

D Occlusal M

Lingual

Mesial

Distal

Buccal

D Occlusal M

Lingual

Mesial

Distal

Mandibular Left Third Molar

CHARACTERISTICS:

Universal Number: #17 **International Number:** #38
Eruption: 17-21
Root completion: 18-25
General crown features: Occlusal table with marginal ridges and cusps with tips, inclined planes, ridges, grooves, fossae, pits
Specific crown features: Smaller crown than second
Height of Contour: Buccal: cervical third; Lingual: middle third
Mesial contact: Cervical third
Distal contact: None
Distinguishing right from left: Wider buccolingually on mesial than on distal
General root features: Two roots
Specific root features: Fused roots, irregularly curved, with sharp apices

Mandibular Left Second Molar

CHARACTERISTICS:

Universal Number: #18 **International Number:** #37
Eruption: 11-13
Root completion: 14-15
General crown features: Occlusal table with marginal ridges and cusps with tips, inclined planes, ridges, grooves, fossae, and pits
Specific crown features: Smaller crown than first. Four cusps with cross-shaped groove pattern
Height of Contour: Buccal: cervical third; Lingual: middle third
Mesial contact: Middle third
Distal contact: Middle third
Distinguishing right from left: Difference in height of contour for buccal and lingual from each proximal surface and wider on mesial than distal
General root features: Two roots
Specific root features: Furcations closer to CEJ. Root trunks and root concavities. Less divergent roots

Mandibular Left First Molar

CHARACTERISTICS:

Universal Number: #19 **International Number:** #36
Eruption: 6-7
Root completion: 9-10
General crown features: Occlusal table with marginal ridges and cusps with tips, inclined planes, ridges, grooves, fossae, and pits
Specific crown features: First permanent tooth to erupt. Widest crown mesiodistally of dentition. Five cusps with Y-shaped groove pattern. Buccal groove possibly ending in buccal pit
Height of Contour: Buccal: cervical third; Lingual: middle third
Mesial contact: Junction of occlusal and middle thirds
Distal contact: Junction of occlusal and middle thirds
Distinguishing right from left: Distal cusp is smallest with sharp cusp
General root features: Two roots
Specific root features: Furcations well removed from CEJ. Root trunks and root concavities. Divergent roots

Mandibular Left Second Premolar (Three-Cusp Type)

CHARACTERISTICS:

Universal Number: #20 **International Number:** #35
Eruption: 11-12
Root completion: 13-14
General crown features: Occlusal table with marginal ridges and cusps with tips, ridges, inclined planes, grooves, fossae, pits. Buccal ridge
Specific crown features: Larger than first. Usually three cusps with Y-shaped groove pattern or two cusps with H or U-shaped groove pattern. Increased supplemental grooves
Height of Contour: Buccal: cervical third; Lingual: middle third
Mesial contact: Just cervical to junction of occlusal and middle thirds
Distal contact: Just cervical to junction of occlusal and middle thirds
Distinguishing right from left: Distal marginal ridge more cervically located with more occlusal surface visible from distal view
General root features: Single root
Specific root features: Oval or elliptical on cervical cross section. Proximal root concavities

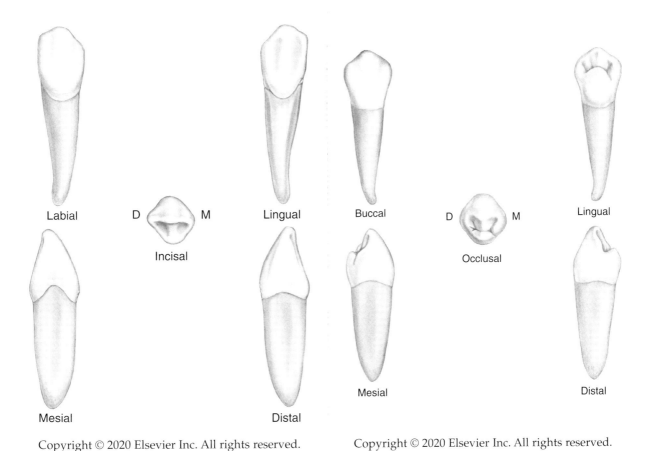

Labial

D Incisal M

Lingual

Mesial

Distal

Buccal

D Occlusal M

Lingual

Mesial

Distal

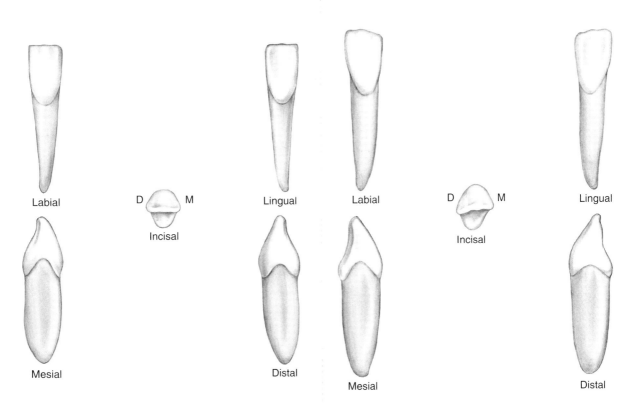

Labial

D Incisal M

Lingual

Mesial

Distal

Labial

D Incisal M

Lingual

Mesial

Distal

Mandibular Left First Premolar

CHARACTERISTICS:

Universal Number: #21 **International Number:** #34
Eruption: 10-12
Root completion: 12-13
General crown features: Occlusal table with marginal ridges and cusps with tips, ridges, inclined planes, grooves, fossae, pits
Specific crown features: Smaller than second. Smaller lingual cusp of two cusps. Mesial surface features. Buccal ridge
Height of Contour: Buccal: cervical third; Lingual: middle third
Mesial contact: Just cervical to junction of occlusal and middle thirds
Distal contact: Just cervical to junction of occlusal and middle thirds
Distinguishing right from left: Shorter mesial cusp slope than distal cusp slope, with mesial surface features: deeper mesial CEJ curvature and mesiolingual groove
General root features: Single root
Specific root features: Oval or elliptical on cervical cross section. Proximal root concavities

Mandibular Left Canine

CHARACTERISTICS:

Universal Number: #22 **International Number:** #33
Eruption: 9-10
Root completion: 12-14
General crown features: Single cusp with tip, slopes, labial ridge, cingulum, lingual ridge, marginal ridges, lingual fossae
Specific crown features: Longest tooth in arch. Less pronounced lingual surface. Less sharp cusp tip
Height of contour: Labial: cervical third; Lingual: middle third
Mesial contact: Incisal third
Distal contact: Junction of incisal and middle thirds
Distinguishing right from left: Shorter mesial cusp slope than distal cusp slope, with more pronounced mesial CEJ curvature. More cervical contact on distal. Shorter and rounder distal outline than mesial outline on labial view, with a shorter mesial slope than distal cusp slope
General root features: Long thick single root
Specific root features: Oval on cervical cross section. Proximal root concavities with developmental depressions on mesial and distal giving tooth double-rooted appearance. Pointed apex

Mandibular Left Lateral Incisor

CHARACTERISTICS:

Universal Number: #23 **International Number:** #32
Eruption: 7-8
Root completion: 10
General crown features: Incisal ridge, incisal angles, cingulum, marginal ridges, lingual fossa
Specific crown features: Like larger mandibular central. Not symmetric. Appears twisted distally. Small distally placed cingulum with mesial marginal ridge longer than distal marginal ridge
Height of contour: Cervical third
Mesial contact: Incisal third
Distal contact: Incisal third
Distinguishing right from left: Sharper mesioincisal angle and rounder distoincisal angle. More pronounced mesial CEJ curvature
General root features: Single root
Specific root features: Elliptical on cervical cross section. Root is longer than crown. Pronounced proximal root concavities can give double-rooted appearance

Mandibular Left Central Incisor

CHARACTERISTICS:

Universal Number: #24 **International Number:** #31
Eruption: 6-7
Root completion: 9
General crown features: Incisal ridge, incisal angles, cingulum, marginal ridges, lingual fossa
Specific crown features: Smallest and simplest tooth. Symmetric. Small centered cingulum, with less pronounced marginal ridges and lingual fossa
Height of contour: Cervical third
Mesial contact: Incisal third
Distal contact: Incisal third
Distinguishing right from left: Sharper mesioincisal angle and rounder distoincisal angle. More pronounced mesial CEJ curvature
General root features: Single root
Specific root features: Elliptical on cervical cross section. Root longer than crown. Pronounced proximal root concavities can give double-rooted appearance

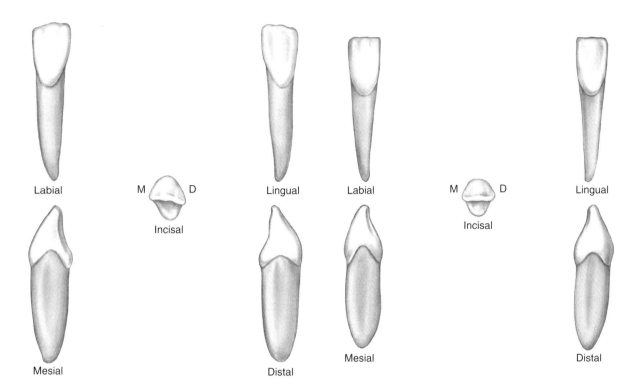

Labial

M ⌣ D
Incisal

Lingual

Labial

M ⌣ D
Incisal

Lingual

Mesial

Distal

Mesial

Distal

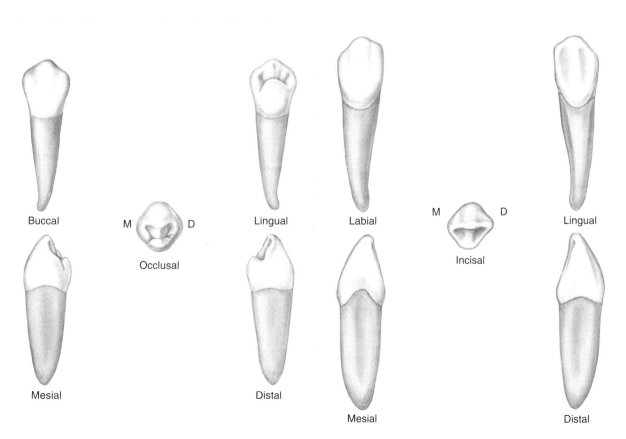

Buccal

M ⌣ D
Occlusal

Lingual

Labial

M ⌣ D
Incisal

Lingual

Mesial

Distal

Mesial

Distal

Mandibular Right Central Incisor

CHARACTERISTICS:

Universal Number: #25 **International Number:** #41
Eruption: 6-7
Root completion: 9
General crown features: Incisal ridge, incisal angles, cingulum, marginal ridges, lingual fossa
Specific crown features: Smallest and simplest tooth. Symmetric. Small centered cingulum, with less pronounced marginal ridges and lingual fossa
Height of contour: Cervical third
Mesial contact: Incisal third
Distal contact: Incisal third
Distinguishing right from left: Sharper mesioincisal angle and rounder distoincisal angle. More pronounced mesial CEJ curvature
General root features: Single root
Specific root features: Elliptical on cervical cross section. Root longer than crown. Pronounced proximal root concavities can give double-rooted appearance

Mandibular Right Lateral Incisor

CHARACTERISTICS:

Universal Number: #26 **International Number:** #42
Eruption: 7-8
Root completion: 10
General crown features: Incisal ridge, incisal angles, cingulum, marginal ridges, lingual fossa
Specific crown features: Like larger mandibular central. Not symmetric. Appears twisted distally. Small distally placed cingulum with mesial marginal ridge longer than distal marginal ridge
Height of contour: Cervical third
Mesial contact: Incisal third
Distal contact: Incisal third
Distinguishing right from left: Sharper mesioincisal angle and rounder distoincisal angle. More pronounced mesial CEJ curvature
General root features: Single root
Specific root features: Elliptical on cervical cross section. Root longer than crown. Proximal root concavities can give double-rooted appearance

Mandibular Right Canine

CHARACTERISTICS:

Universal Number: #27 **International Number:** #43
Eruption: 9-10
Root completion: 12-14
General crown features: Single cusp with tip, slopes, labial ridge, cingulum, lingual ridge, marginal ridges, lingual fossae
Specific crown features: Longest tooth in arch. Less pronounced lingual surface. Less sharp cusp tip
Height of contour: Labial: cervical third; Lingual: middle third
Mesial contact: Incisal third
Distal contact: Junction of incisal and middle thirds
Distinguishing right from left: Shorter mesial cusp slope than distal cusp slope with more pronounced mesial CEJ curvature. More cervical contact on distal. Shorter and rounder distal outline than mesial outline on labial view with a shorter mesial slope than distal slope
General root features: Long thick single root
Specific root features: Oval on cervical cross section. Proximal root concavities with developmental depressions on mesial and distal giving tooth double-rooted appearance. Pointed apex

Mandibular Right First Premolar

CHARACTERISTICS:

Universal Number: #28 **International Number:** #44
Eruption: 10-12
Root completion: 12-13
General crown features: Occlusal table with marginal ridges and cusps with tips, ridges, inclined planes, grooves, fossae, pits.
Specific crown features: Smaller than second. Smaller lingual cusp of two cusps. Mesial surface features. Buccal ridge
Height of Contour: Buccal: cervical third; Lingual: middle third
Mesial contact: Just cervical to junction of occlusal and middle thirds
Distal contact: Just cervical to junction of occlusal and middle thirds
Distinguishing right from left: Shorter mesial cusp slope than distal cusp slope and with mesial surface features: deeper mesial CEJ curvature and mesiolingual groove
General root features: Single root
Specific root features: Oval or elliptical on cervical cross section. Proximal root concavities

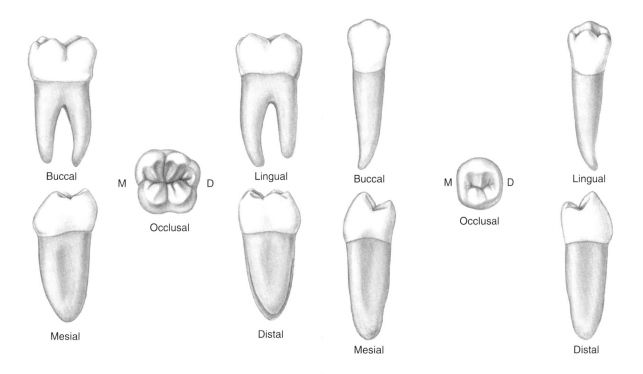

Buccal

M Occlusal D

Lingual

Mesial

Distal

Buccal

M Occlusal D

Lingual

Mesial

Distal

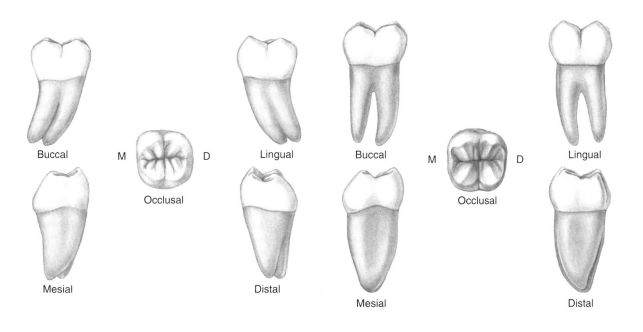

Buccal

M Occlusal D

Lingual

Mesial

Distal

Buccal

M Occlusal D

Lingual

Mesial

Distal

Mandibular Right Second Premolar (Three-Cusp Type)

CHARACTERISTICS:

Universal Number: #29 **International Number:** #45
Eruption: 11-12
Root completion: 13-14
General crown features: Occlusal table with marginal ridges and cusps with tips, ridges, inclined planes, grooves, fossae, pits
Specific crown features: Larger than first. Usually three cusps with Y-shaped groove pattern or two cusps with H- or U-shaped groove pattern. Increased supplemental grooves. Buccal ridge
Height of Contour: Buccal: cervical third; Lingual: middle third
Mesial contact: Just cervical to junction of occlusal and middle thirds
Distal contact: Just cervical to junction of occlusal and middle thirds
Distinguishing right from left: Distal marginal ridge more cervically located with more occlusal surface visible from distal view
General root features: Single root
Specific root features: Oval or elliptical on cervical cross section. Proximal root concavities

Mandibular Right First Molar

CHARACTERISTICS:

Universal Number: #30 **International Number:** #46
Eruption: 6-7
Root completion: 9-10
General crown features: Occlusal table with marginal ridges and cusps with tips, inclined planes, ridges, grooves, fossae, pits
Specific crown features: First permanent tooth to erupt. Widest crown mesiodistally of dentition. Five cusps with Y-shaped groove pattern. Buccal groove possibly ending in buccal pit
Height of Contour: Buccal: cervical third; Lingual: middle third
Mesial contact: Junction of occlusal and middle thirds
Distal contact: Junction of occlusal and middle thirds
Distinguishing right from left: Distal cusp is smallest and has a sharp cusp
General root features: Two roots
Specific root features: Furcations well removed from CEJ. Root trunks and root concavities. Divergent roots

Mandibular Right Second Molar

CHARACTERISTICS:

Universal Number: #31 **International Number:** #47
Eruption: 11-13
Root completion: 14-15
General crown features: Occlusal table with marginal ridges and cusps with tips, inclined planes, ridges, grooves, fossae, pits
Specific crown features: Smaller crown than first. Four cusps with cross-shaped groove pattern
Height of Contour: Buccal: cervical third; Lingual: middle third
Mesial contact: Middle third
Distal contact: Middle third
Distinguishing right from left: Difference in height of contour for buccal and lingual from each proximal surface and wider on mesial than distal
General root features: Two roots
Specific root features: Furcations closer to CEJ. Root trunks and root concavities. Less divergent roots

Mandibular Right Third Molar

CHARACTERISTICS:

Universal Number: #32 **International Number:** #48
Eruption: 17-21
Root completion: 18-25
General crown features: Occlusal table with marginal ridges and cusps with tips, inclined planes, ridges, grooves, fossae, pits
Specific crown features: Smaller crown than second
Height of Contour: Buccal: cervical third; Lingual: middle third
Mesial contact: Cervical third
Distal contact: None
Distinguishing right from left: Wider buccolingually on mesial than on distal
General root features: Two roots
Specific root features: Fused roots. Irregularly curved with sharp apices